Department of Health
National Assembly for Wales
Scottish Executive Health Department
DHSS PS (Northern Ireland)
with the
Public Health Laboratory Service
Communicable Disease Surveillance Centre

HEALTH INFORMATION for OVERSEAS TRAVEL

2nd Edition

2001

LONDON: The Stationery Office

Printed in the United Kingdom for The Stationery Office C900 10/01

Preface

Health Information for Overseas Travel was first issued in 1995 as a companion volume to the well established UK Health Departments' memorandum Immunisation against Infectious Disease (the 'Green Book'). It was well received, especially by doctors and practice nurses giving travel health advice in primary care, and is now commonly referred to as the UK 'Yellow Book'.

Since that first edition, there has been a major increase in the amount of travel-related information available both to health professionals and travellers, in books, the media and via the Internet. The origins and significance of the information are not always clear, however, and the advice may not be consistent with that usually given in the UK.

The aim of this book is therefore still relevant: to provide a concise and authoritative one-stop source of information about the common health risks to travellers and how to reduce them. It is not a statement of Government policy. It is advisory rather than prescriptive, emphasising the need to assess the risks for the individual traveller, while recognising the limitations of the data on which such assessments sometimes have to be made. Risk behaviours are also discussed, and emphasis put on measures travellers themselves can take to protect their health abroad.

Further sources of advice are provided for more specialised problems outside the scope of this book.

We have pleasure in commending the book, and thank the editors, Dr Gil Lea of the Public Health Laboratory Service Communicable Disease Surveillance Centre, and Dr Jane Leese from the Department of Health, for their work in updating the information for this edition.

Professor Liam Donaldson   Dr Ruth Hall

Dr Mac Armstrong   Dr Henrietta Campbell

Chief Medical Officers

Contributors

The following have kindly contributed to the revision of this book:

Dr Barbara Bannister   Dr Mary Ramsay
Dr Ronald Behrens   Rosemary Tucker
Prof David Bradley   Dr Eric Walker
Dr Peter Chiodini   Dr John Watson

Thanks are also due to the medical staff at the Department of Health and the Public Health Laboratory Service, particulary Dr B Evans, Dr A Nicoll and Dr Carol Joseph who read and commented on the text, Dr N Byrne, Dr C Conlon and Diabetes UK.

Emma Wilbraham, Jeff Porter and Julie Pettman masterminded production. Without them this revision would never have seen the light of day.

Thanks are also extended to the original contributors Dr A Bulman, B Carroll, Prof R Cartwright, Dr C Dow, Dr R Fairhurst, Dr J Porter, Dr J Sergeant and Prof D Warrell. Much of the information on disease risks is reproduced, with their kind permission, from the World Health Organization booklet *International Travel and Health – Vaccination Requirements and Health Advice* 2001, to which acknowledgement is made. Our thanks in particular go to the editor Mary Vallanjon.

Comments, corrections and suggestions for improving future editions of this publication, are welcome (see page 147).

Dr Gil Lea   Dr Jane Leese
Public Health Laboratory Service   *Department of Health*
Communicable Disease
Surveillance Centre

Editors

Contents

Maps

Introduction – how to use this book

1.1   This book starts with descriptions by continental group of the disease and health risks most likely to be encountered by travellers, with recommendations for their prevention. For ease of reference the section for each continental group follows the same format:

1. A list of the countries covered in the section

2. Disease risks:
   - Food and water-borne diseases
   - Malaria
   - Other arthropod-borne diseases
   - Diseases of close association
   - Sexually transmitted and blood-borne diseases
   - Other hazards

3. Recommendations which apply to all countries in the group

4. Country by country variations for immunisations, including yellow fever vaccination requirements, and recommendations for malaria chemoprophylaxis. (It follows that countries not mentioned individually do not vary from the general advice.)

1.2   Countries have been grouped with those for which similar general advice may apply within recognisable geographical areas. For example, the term 'Indian Sub-continent' is used rather than 'Middle South Asia', which may be less readily recognised. These groupings have no political significance and are entirely pragmatic.

1.3   The book is intended as a practical handbook and not a textbook. The diseases listed are not exhaustive – those which are mainly of importance to the indigenous population and unlikely to afflict travellers are largely omitted. Those who require further detail are referred to the bibliography at the end of the book.

1.4   While the recommendations for each continental group in Chapter 3 are about immunisations and malaria chemoprophylaxis, it must be remembered that most health problems affecting travellers are not vaccine preventable. Advice about accident and injury prevention, food and water hygiene, protection against insect bites and sexual health may be equally important. These subjects are dealt with in the succeeding chapters.

1.5   It should also be remembered that diseases which are common at home, such as respiratory illness and cardiovascular diseases, may occur during travel. Travellers should ensure that they obtain medical insurance to cover these and other contingencies. Any prescription medicines should be clearly labelled, preferably in the original container with the chemist's label, and carried in hand luggage. In situations where the possession of even prescription drugs might be queried, or if the drugs themselves are unusual or need to be injected, it is advisable to carry a doctor's letter to confirm they are needed.

1.6   Recommendations for immunisations assume that routine immunisations are up to date (see Chapter 8 and the UK Health Departments' memorandum Immunisation against Infectious Disease for further details).

1.7   Since most decisions about vaccines for travel involve consideration of the risk to the individual traveller, experts may disagree on the detail of recommendations and travellers may receive conflicting information. The advice in this book is based on consensus with the aim of reducing such confusion, but it cannot encompass every circumstance. It is not a statement of Government policy.

1.8   The elimination of poliomyelitis in certain areas may result in a debate as to whether immunisation is still indicated. It is still recommended that all travellers have been immunised against polio; this provides protection for the individual traveller, but also, importantly, prevents visitors reintroducing wild polio virus into countries free of polio. However, booster doses are advised for fewer countries.

1.9   The rabies free areas listed are provided as guidance for decisions about pre-exposure prophylaxis. In occasional circumstances, post exposure prophylaxis could be indicated for additional areas, for example when the animal involved could have been imported, and specialist advice should always be sought.

1.10   The international yellow fever vaccination certificate requirements quoted are based on those published by the World Health Organization in the 2001 edition of *International Travel and Health*. This is revised annually.

What's new: changes since the last edition

1.11   A number of changes have been made since the first edition of *Health Information for Overseas Travel*:

1. Disease risks and advice on immunisations and malaria chemoprophylaxis have been updated.

2. Polio boosters are no longer recommended for those travelling to the

Americas, including South and Central America and the Caribbean, so long as individuals have had a primary course of polio vaccine during their lifetime (see 1.8 above).

3. Diphtheria/tetanus combined vaccine is generally now recommended where tetanus immunisation is indicated (see 8.4).

4. The typhoid immunisation advice better reflects the recent epidemiology of this disease.

5. Chapters 6 (Prevention of malaria) and 8 (Immunisation for overseas travel) have been substantially revised and updated. Information on malaria is based on the 2001 *Guidelines for malaria prevention in travellers from the United Kingdom.*

6. Several new vaccines have become available, including a number of combined vaccines. A new conjugate meningococcal C vaccine has now been introduced into the routine childhood immunisation schedule but for travel meningococcal A&C vaccine is the usually recommended vaccine (see 8.4.4).

7. Three new chapters have been included: 'Arthropod-borne diseases' (Chapter 7), 'Medical considerations for the journey' (Chapter 13) and 'Travellers with pre-existing medical conditions' (Chapter 14).

8. The list of yellow fever vaccination centres has been removed due to the constant changes. These are now available from:

England
Mrs Sue Doran
Department of Health
Room 601a
Skipton House
80 London Road
London SE1 6LH

N Ireland
Mr Michael Kelly
Public Health Branch
Department of Health and Social Services
and Public Safety
Room C4.15
Castle Buildings
Stormont
Belfast BT4 3PP

Tel: 0207 972 5047
Email: Sue.doran@doh.gsi.gov.uk

Tel: 02890 522118
Email: Michael.kelly2@dhsspsni.gov.uk

Scotland

Mr Charles Hodgson
Public Health Policy Unit Branch 1
Scottish Executive Health Department
3E (South)
St Andrews House
Regent Road
Edinburgh EH1 3DG

Tel: 0131 244 2501
Email:
Charles.hodgson@scotland.gov.uk

Wales

Miss Catherine Cody
Public Health Division
National Assembly for Wales
Cathays Park
Cardiff CF10 3NQ

Tel: 02920 823395
Email: Catherine.cody@
wales.gsi.gov.uk

9. New web site addresses and references have been included.

1.12 This reference book is available on the Internet.

1.13 Information on recent disease outbreaks can be found on the Department of Health website at http://www.doh.gov.uk/hat/emerg.htm and CEEFAX/ PRESTEL.

List of countries by continental group

Please note that countries have been grouped with those for which similar general advice may apply within recognisable geographic areas. For example, the term 'Indian Subcontinent' is used rather than 'Middle South Asia' which may be less readily recognised by users. These groupings are entirely pragmatic and have no political significance.

Europe, including Cyprus and countries of the former USSR

Albania	Germany	Norway
Andorra	Gibraltar	Poland
Armenia	Greece	Portugal (with the
Austria	Hungary	Azores and Madeira)
Azerbaijan	Iceland	Romania
Belarus	Ireland	Russia
Belgium	Italy	San Marino
Bosnia & Herzegovina	Kazakhstan	Slovakia
Bulgaria	Kyrgyzstan	Slovenia
Croatia	Latvia	Spain (with the Canary
Cyprus	Liechtenstein	Islands)
Czech Republic	Lithuania	Sweden
Denmark (with the	Luxembourg	Switzerland
Faroe Islands)	Macedonia	Tajikistan
Estonia	Malta	Turkmenistan
Finland	Moldova	Ukraine
France	Monaco	Uzbekistan
Georgia	Netherlands	Yugoslavia (including
		Kosovo, Montenegro
		and Serbia)

North America, Australia and New Zealand

Australia	Greenland	United States of
Bermuda	New Zealand	America (with Hawaii)
Canada	Saint Pierre and Miquelon	

Central America

Belize	Guatemala	Nicaragua
Costa Rica	Honduras	Panama
El Salvador	Mexico	

The Caribbean

Anguilla	Dominican Republic	Saint Kitts and Nevis Antigua
and Barbuda	Grenada	Saint Lucia
Aruba	Guadeloupe	Saint Vincent and the
Bahamas	Haiti	Grenadines
Barbados	Jamaica	Trinidad and Tobago
British Virgin Islands	Martinique	Turks and Caicos Islands
Cayman Islands	Montserrat	Virgin Islands (USA)
Cuba	Netherlands Antilles	
Dominica	Puerto Rico	

Tropical South America

Bolivia	French Guiana	Surinam
Brazil	Guyana	Venezuela (including
Colombia	Paraguay	Marguerita Island)
Ecuador (including	Peru	
Galapagos)		

Temperate South America

Argentina	Falkland Islands	Uruguay
Chile		

Northern Africa and the Middle East, including Afghanistan and Turkey

Afghanistan	Jordan	Saudi Arabia
Algeria	Kuwait	Syria
Bahrain	Lebanon	Tunisia
Egypt	Libya	Turkey
Iran	Morocco	United Arab Emirates
Iraq	Oman	Yemen
Israel	Qatar	

Sub-Saharan and Southern Africa

Angola	Ghana	Saint Helena
Benin	Guinea	Sao Tome and Principe
Botswana	Guinea-Bissau	Senegal
Burkina Faso	Ivory Coast	Seychelles
Burundi	Kenya	Sierra Leone
Cameroon	Lesotho	Somalia
Cape Verde	Liberia	South Africa
Central African Republic	Madagascar	Sudan
Chad	Malawi	Swaziland
Comoros	Mali	Tanzania (including
Congo	Mauritania	Zanzibar)

Democratic Republic of Congo (formerly Zaire)
Djibouti
Equatorial Guinea
Eritrea
Ethiopia
Gabon
Gambia

Mauritius
Mayotte
Mozambique
Namibia
Niger
Nigeria
Reunion
Rwanda

Togo
Uganda
Zaire (see Democratic Republic of Congo)
Zambia
Zanzibar (see Tanzania)
Zimbabwe

Indian Subcontinent

Bangladesh
Bhutan
India

Maldives
Nepal
Pakistan

Sri Lanka

South East Asia and the Far East

Borneo (see Indonesia and Malaysia)
Brunei Darussalam
Burma (see Myanmar)
Cambodia
China
East Timor
Hong Kong (see China)
Indonesia (including Bali and Southern Borneo)

Japan
Korea
Laos
Macao (See China)
Malaysia (Penisular Malaysia and Northern Borneo, including Sarawak and Sabah)

Mongolia
Myanmar
Philippines
Singapore
Taiwan
Thailand
Tibet (see China)
Vietnam

Pacific Islands

American Samoa
Cook Islands
Easter Island
Fiji
French Polynesia (Tahiti)
Guam
Kiribati
Marshall Islands

Micronesia (Federated States of)
Nauru
New Caledonia
Niue
Palau
Papua New Guinea
Samoa

Solomon Islands
Tokelau
Tonga
Trust Territory of the Pacific Islands
Tuvalu
Vanuatu
Wallis and Futuna Islands

3 Disease risks and recommendations by continental group and country

3.1 Europe, including Cyprus and countries of the former USSR

(Albania, Andorra, Armenia, Austria, Azerbaijan, Belarus, Belgium, Bosnia and Herzegovina, Bulgaria, Croatia, Cyprus, Czech Republic, Denmark (with the Faroe Islands), Estonia, Finland, France, Georgia, Germany, Gibraltar, Greece, Hungary, Iceland, Ireland, Italy, Kazakhstan, Kyrgyzstan, Latvia, Liechtenstein, Lithuania, Luxembourg, Macedonia, Malta, Moldova, Monaco, Netherlands, Norway, Poland, Portugal (with the Azores and Madeira), Romania, Russia, San Marino, Slovakia, Slovenia, Spain (with the Canary Islands), Sweden, Switzerland, Tajikistan, Turkmenistan, Ukraine, Uzbekistan, Yugoslavia (including Kosovo, Montenegro and Serbia)

3.1.1 Disease risks

For much of the area communicable diseases are unlikely to prove a hazard greater than in the UK. The risks may be higher in parts of Eastern Europe, but lack of information makes risk assessment difficult.

Food and water-borne diseases (bacillary dysentery, other diarrhoeas, and typhoid) are most likely to occur in the south-eastern and south-western parts of the area, especially in summer and autumn. The incidence of certain food-borne diseases, eg salmonella and campylobacter infections, is increasing in some countries. Hepatitis A is commoner in the eastern European countries.

Malaria is confined to small foci in Armenia, Azerbaijan, Georgia, Tajikistan and Turkmenistan.

Other arthropod-borne diseases (see Chapter 7) occur of which the most common are:
- Tick-borne encephalitis – mainly in forests and surrounding areas in central and eastern Europe and Scandinavia and across the former USSR to the Pacific coast.
- Lyme disease
- Tick-borne typhus – in Siberia and the Mediterranean
- Japanese encephalitis – in a small area in the far eastern maritime areas of the former USSR neighbouring China
- Murine typhus (endemic) – sporadic cases occur in some countries bordering the Mediterranean littoral

Map to show how countries are grouped for pragmatic reasons and the order (by number) in which they appear in the text in Chapter 3.

1 Europe
2 North America, Australia and New Zealand
3 Central America
4 The Caribbean
5 Tropical South America
6 Temperate South America
7 North Africa and Middle East
8 Sub-Saharan and Southern Africa
9 Indian Subcontinent
10 South East Asia and the Far East
11 Pacific islands

- West Nile Fever – cases sometimes occur in Mediterranean and eastern European countries
- Cutaneous and visceral leishmaniasis and sand fly fever reported from Southern Europe
- Leishmania/HIV co-infection reported from France, Greece, Italy
- Tularaemia in parts of continental Europe.
- Louse-borne relapsing fever in Turkey and areas of the former USSR.
- Tick-borne relapsing fever – foci in Portugal and Spain

Diseases of close association:

- In recent years, Azerbaijan, Belarus, Russia and Ukraine have experienced extensive epidemics of diphtheria. Cases of diphtheria, mostly imported from these three countries, have also been reported in neighbouring countries (Estonia, Finland, Latvia, Lithuania, Poland, the Republic of Moldova).
- All countries are making intense efforts to eradicate polio, and the risk of infection in most countries is very low.
- Tuberculosis rates are increasing in parts of eastern Europe and the former USSR, including drug resistant disease.

Sexually transmitted and blood-borne infections:
Hepatitis B is generally of low prevalence; prevalence higher in the eastern and southern parts of the region. HIV is predominantly in high risk groups, but the risk of all STIs, particularly for young travellers, should not be forgotten.

Other hazards could include:

- Legionnaires' disease – both sporadic cases and clusters of cases associated with holiday hotels and apartments continue to be reported in returning travellers.
- Leptospirosis.
- Rodent-borne haemorrhagic fever with renal syndrome (Hanta virus infection) is now recognised as occurring in some areas in this region.
- Rabies is endemic in wild animals (particularly foxes) in rural areas of northern and eastern Europe and in most countries of southern Europe apart from: Cyprus, Faroe Islands, Finland, Greece, Iceland, Ireland, mainland Italy (except the northern and eastern borders), mainland Norway, mainland Spain (except the N African coast), Sweden, Gibraltar, Malta, Portugal and Monaco. However, the latter country has land borders with France (see 1.9).

Parts of northern Europe can be extremely cold in winter.

3.1.2 Recommendations for immunisations and malaria chemoprophylaxis (see later chapters for general health precautions)

FOR ALL COUNTRIES

Check routine immunisations including tetanus.

For immunisation recommendations for poliomyelitis boosters, hepatitis A and typhoid please see the country by country guide below, noting that immunisation against typhoid and/or hepatitis A may be less important for short stays in standard business or tourist conditions. For polio, see also paragraph 1.8.

Those walking or camping in late spring and summer in rural parts of central and eastern Europe (including the former USSR) and Scandinavia, are at increased risk of tick-borne encephalitis – consider immunisation (see also Chapter 7).

For long stay visitors to eastern Europe and the former USSR consider immunisation against diphtheria and hepatitis B, and check BCG status; for those going to live or work with local people, a diphtheria booster may be considered even for shorter stays if the last dose was more than 10 years ago. For remote areas out of reach of medical attention, possibly also consider rabies vaccine.

3.1.3 Country by country variations and malaria chemoprophylaxis:

Albania
Yellow fever vaccination certificate **required** from travellers over one year old coming from infected areas.

Immunisation against poliomyelitis and hepatitis A usually advised.

Armenia
Immunisation against hepatitis A usually advised.

Malaria risk: *P.vivax* malaria focally in Ararat Valley, from June to October, outside tourist areas.

Recommended prophylaxis: for the risk area only, chloroquine.

Austria
Tick-borne encephalitis vaccine in certain circumstances (see 7.4).

Azerbaijan
Immunisation against hepatitis A and typhoid usually advised.

Malaria risk: *P.vivax* malaria focally, from June to October.

Recommended prophylaxis: chloroquine.

Belarus
Immunisation against hepatitis A usually advised.

Tick-borne encephalitis vaccine in certain circumstances (see 7.4).

Bosnia
Immunisation against hepatitis A usually advised.

Bulgaria
Immunisation against hepatitis A usually advised.

Croatia
Immunisation against hepatitis A usually advised.

Tick-borne encephalitis vaccine in certain circumstances (see 7.4).

Czech Republic
Immunisation against hepatitis A usually advised.

Tick-borne encephalitis vaccine in certain circumstances (see 7.4).

Estonia
Tick-borne encephalitis vaccine in certain circumstances (see 7.4).

Georgia
Immunisation against hepatitis A usually advised.

Malaria risk: *P.vivax* malaria focally in rural areas in the south-east, June to October.

Recommended prophylaxis: for those areas only, chloroquine.

Germany
Tick-borne encephalitis vaccine in certain circumstances (see 7.4).

Greece
Yellow fever vaccination certificate **required** from travellers over six months old coming from infected areas.

Hepatitis A immunisation occasionally advised, eg for those on extensive backpacking holidays where food hygiene might be in doubt.

Herzegovina
Immunisation against hepatitis A usually advised.

Hungary
Tick-borne encephalitis vaccine in certain circumstances (see 7.4).

Kazakhstan
Yellow fever vaccination certificate **required** from travellers coming from infected areas.

Immunisation against poliomyelitis, hepatitis A and typhoid usually advised.

Kyrgyzstan
Immunisation against poliomyelitis, hepatitis A and typhoid usually advised.

Latvia
Tick-borne encephalitis vaccine in certain circumstances (see 7.4).

Lithuania
Tick-borne encephalitis vaccine in certain circumstances (see 7.4).

Macedonia
Immunisation against hepatitis A usually advised.

Malta
Yellow fever vaccination certificate **required** from travellers over nine months old coming from infected areas. (If indicated on epidemiological grounds, infants under nine months of age coming from infected areas are subject to isolation or surveillance).

Moldova
Immunisation against hepatitis A usually advised.

Poland
Tick-borne encephalitis vaccine in certain circumstances (see 7.4).

Portugal, with the Azores and Madeira
Yellow fever vaccination certificate required from travellers over one year old coming from infected areas and arriving in or bound for the Azores and Madeira. No certificate is required from passengers in transit at Funchal, Porto Santo and Santa Maria.

Hepatitis A immunisation occasionally advised, eg for those on extensive backpacking holidays where food hygiene might be in doubt.

Romania
Immunisation against hepatitis A usually advised.

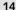

Russia

Immunisation against poliomyelitis, hepatitis A and typhoid usually advised for areas east of the Urals.

Japanese encephalitis and Russian spring summer encephalitis – consider immunisation against JE for far eastern maritime areas, south of Khabarousk, July–September.

Tick-borne encephalitis vaccine in certain circumstances (see 7.4).

Slovakia

Immunisation against hepatitis A usually advised.

Tick-borne encephalitis vaccine in certain circumstances (see 7.4).

Slovenia

Immunisation against hepatitis A usually advised.

Tick-borne encephalitis vaccine in certain circumstances (see 7.4).

Tajikistan

Immunisation against poliomyelitis, hepatitis A and typhoid usually advised.

Malaria risk: malaria (mostly *P.vivax*) patchily distributed, June to October.

Recommended prophylaxis: chloroquine.

Turkmenistan

Immunisation against poliomyelitis, hepatitis A and typhoid usually advised.

Malaria risk: *P.vivax* from June to October in south-eastern region.

Recommended prophylaxis: in the risk area, chloroquine.

Ukraine

Immunisation against hepatitis A usually advised.

Tick-borne encephalitis vaccine in certain circumstances (see 7.4).

Uzbekistan

Immunisation against poliomyelitis, hepatitis A and typhoid usually advised.

Yugoslavia

Immunisation against hepatitis A usually advised.

3.2   North America, Australia and New Zealand

(Australia, Bermuda, Canada, Greenland, New Zealand, Saint Pierre and Miquelon and the United States of America (with Hawaii))

3.2.1   Disease risks

Communicable diseases are unlikely to prove a hazard greater than that found in the UK.

Malaria is not endemic in these areas.

Other arthropod-borne diseases (see Chapter 7) include various strains of viral encephalitis in some rural areas of Australia (eg Ross River fever) and USA (eg West Nile Virus, St Louis encephalitis).

- Japanese encephalitis confined to islands of Torres Strait and sporadic cases at Cape York Peninsula.
- Lyme disease is endemic in north-eastern, mid-Atlantic and upper Midwest USA, with occasional cases reported from the Pacific north-west.
- Rocky Mountain spotted fever and tularaemia occur occasionally in N America.
- Dengue fever has occurred in northern Australia in recent years; it is endemic in Hawaii and has occurred in South USA.
- Plague in USA.
- Tick-borne relapsing fever in west USA and west Canada.
- Tick and scrub typhus in Queensland, Australia.

Diseases of close association:
- Poliomyelitis has been eliminated in the Americas, Australia and New Zealand.
- Tuberculosis predominantly in certain high risk groups (as in the UK).

Sexually transmitted and blood-borne infections:
- Hepatitis B highly prevalent in certain indigenous groups in N. Canada, Alaska, Greenland, Australia and New Zealand.
- HIV predominantly in high risk groups.

Other hazards could include:

In N. America – leptospirosis, hantavirus (mainly in the western states of the USA and SW provinces of Canada); rabies in wildlife (including bats); poisonous snakes; poison ivy, poison oak; very low temperatures in the north in winter.

In Australia and New Zealand – Corals and jelly fish and spines of poisonous fish during sea bathing; snakes and venomous spiders in Australia. Insectivorous and fruit-eating bats in Australia have been found to harbour a rabies-related virus. Heat in northern and central Australia.

3.2.2 Recommendations for immunisations and malaria chemoprophylaxis (see later chapters for general health precautions)

FOR ALL COUNTRIES

Check routine immunisations including tetanus.

3.2.3 Country by country variations:

Australia

Yellow fever vaccination certificate required from travellers over one year of age entering Australia within six days of having stayed overnight or longer in an infected country, as listed in the WHO Weekly Epidemiological Record.

Japanese encephalitis – consider vaccination only for those going to live or work in Torres Strait Islands.

USA

Proof of immunisation against diphtheria, measles, poliomyelitis and rubella is now universally required for entry into school. Schools in most states also require proof of immunisation against tetanus (49 states), pertussis (44 states), mumps (43 states) and hepatitis B (26 states). Some universities and schools may ask for varicella immunisation.

3.3   Central America

(Belize, Costa Rica, El Salvador, Guatemala, Honduras, Mexico, Nicaragua, Panama)

3.3.1   Disease risks

Food and water-borne diseases including amoebic and bacillary dysentry, other diarrhoeal diseases and typhoid fever are common throughout the area. Hepatitis A occurs throughout the area and hepatitis E has been reported in Mexico. Helminth infections are also common. All countries except Panama have reported cholera in recent years.

Malaria present in all countries – see individual entries below

Other arthropod-borne diseases (see Chapter 7):
- Yellow fever – the South American endemic zone extends into Panama
- Cutaneous and mucocutaneous leishmaniasis in all countries
- Visceral leishmaniasis – El Salvador, Guatemala, Honduras, Mexico and Nicaragua
- Onchocerciasis (river blindness) in two small foci in the south of Mexico and four dispersed foci in Guatemala
- American trypanosomiasis (Chagas' disease) in localised foci in rural areas in all countries
- Dengue fever and Venezuelan equine encephalitis may occur in all countries
- Rocky Mountain spotted fever.

Diseases of close association:
- In 1994, an international commission certified the eradication of endemic wild poliovirus from the Americas. Ongoing surveillance in formerly endemic Central and South American countries confirms that poliovirus transmission remains interrupted.
- Tuberculosis endemic.

Sexually transmitted and blood-borne infections:
Hepatitis B of low prevalence in most countries (intermediate prevalence in Guatemala and Honduras); HIV endemic throughout the area.

Other hazards could include:
- Leptospirosis.
- Rabies in animals (usually dogs and bats).
- Snakes and scorpions in some areas.

3.3.2 Recommendations for immunisations and malaria chemoprophylaxis (see later chapters for general health precautions)

FOR ALL COUNTRIES

Check routine immunisations including tetanus.

Immunisation against hepatitis A and typhoid generally advised.

For longer stays, consider immunisation against diphtheria, hepatitis B and check BCG status; for longer rural travel, out of reach of medical attention, consider immunisation against rabies.

3.3.3 Country by country variations and malaria chemoprophylaxis:

Belize

Yellow fever vaccination certificate required from travellers coming from infected areas.

Malaria risk (predominantly *P.vivax*) throughout the year.

Recommended prophylaxis: chloroquine.

Costa Rica

Malaria risk (almost exclusively *P.vivax*) throughout the year in rural areas below 700m in Alajuela, Guanacaste, Limon and Heredia provinces.

Recommended prophylaxis: for the rural areas above only, chloroquine.

El Salvador

Yellow fever vaccination certificate required from travellers over six months of age coming from infected areas.

Malaria risk (almost exclusively *P.vivax*) throughout the year in Santa Ana province.

Recommended prophylaxis: for the risk area, chloroquine.

Guatemala

Yellow fever vaccination certificate required from travellers over one year of age coming from countries with infected areas.

Malaria risk (predominantly *P.vivax*) throughout the year below 1,500m in several Departments.

Recommended prophylaxis: chloroquine.

Honduras

Yellow fever vaccination certificate required from travellers coming from infected areas.

Malaria risk (predominantly *P.vivax*) throughout the year in most areas.

Recommended prophylaxis: chloroquine.

Mexico

Malaria risk (almost exclusively *P.vivax*) throughout the year largely in rural areas. There is a significant risk of transmission in the states of: Campeche, Chiapas, Guerrero, Michoacan, Oaxaca, Quintana Roo, Sinaloa and Tabasco and moderate risk in the states of Chichuahua, Durango, Hidalgo, Jalisco, Nayarit, Sonora and Veracruz.

Recommended prophylaxis: for the risk areas, chloroquine; in other areas none but bear in mind the remote possibility of malaria.

Nicaragua

Yellow fever vaccination certificate required from travellers over one year of age coming from infected areas.

Malaria risk (predominantly *P.vivax*) throughout the year in most areas.

Recommended prophylaxis: chloroquine.

Panama

Yellow fever vaccination certificate recommended for all travellers going to Chepo Darien and San Blas.

Malaria risk (predominantly *P.vivax*) throughout the year in three provinces: Bocas de Toro in the west, and Darien and San Blas in the east where chloroquine resistant *P.falciparum* has been reported. The canal area itself is considered malaria free.

Recommended prophylaxis: for above areas, chloroquine west of the canal; chloroquine plus proguanil east of the canal.

3.4   The Caribbean

(Anguilla, Antigua and Barbuda, Aruba, Bahamas, Barbados, British Virgin Islands, Cayman Islands, Cuba, Dominica, Dominican Republic, Grenada, Guadeloupe, Haiti, Jamaica, Martinique, Montserrat, Netherlands Antilles, Puerto Rico, Saint Kitts and Nevis, Saint Lucia, Saint Vincent and the Grenadines, Trinidad and Tobago, Turks and Caicos Islands, and the Virgin Islands (USA)).

3.4.1   Disease risks

Food and water-borne diseases:
Bacillary and amoebic dysentery are common and hepatitis A reported, particularly in the northern islands. No cholera has been reported in recent years.

Biointoxication may occur from raw or cooked fish or shellfish.

Malaria: only in Haiti and the Dominican Republic

Other arthropod-borne diseases (see Chapter 7):
● Outbreaks of dengue fever and some dengue haemorrhagic fever.
● Diffuse cutaneous leishmaniasis recently reported from Dominican Republic.
● Bancroftian filariasis in Haiti and some other islands.
● Other filariases occasionally found.
● Fasciola hepatica endemic in Cuba.
● Yellow fever reported in wildlife in Trinidad.

Diseases of close association:
● In 1994, an international commission certified the eradication of endemic wild poliovirus from the Americas including the Caribbean. Ongoing surveillance in formerly endemic Central and South American countries confirms that poliovirus transmission remains interrupted, although an outbreak of vaccine-derived poliovirus type 1 occurred in the Dominican Republic and Haiti in July 2000.
● Tuberculosis incidence similar to western Europe, although higher in Haiti and the Dominican Republic.

Sexually transmitted and blood-borne infections:
Hepatitis B of low or intermediate prevalence; HIV endemic.

Other hazards could include:
● Schistosomiasis (bilharziasis) in the Dominican Republic, Guadeloupe, Martinique, Puerto Rico and Saint Lucia; may occur sporadically in other islands.
● Spiny sea urchins, corals and jellyfish, snakes and scorpions.
● Animal rabies, particularly in the mongoose, reported from several islands.

3.4.2 Recommendations for immunisations and malaria chemoprophylaxis (see later chapters for general health precautions)

FOR ALL COUNTRIES

Check routine immunisations including tetanus.

Immunisation against hepatitis A usually advised (less important for short stays in tourist hotels). Immunsation against typhoid occasionally advised for longer stays where food and water hygiene standards may be in doubt.

For longer stays consider immunisation against hepatitis B and diphtheria and check BCG status.

3.4.3 Country by country variations and malaria chemoprophylaxis:

Anguilla, Antigua and Barbuda, Bahamas, Barbados, Dominica
Yellow fever vaccination certificate **required** from travellers over one year of age coming from infected areas.

Dominican Republic
Malaria – low risk throughout the year. Because the malaria is almost exclusively of the more severe falciparum type and still sensitive to chloroquine it is wise for travellers to take prophylaxis.

Recommended prophylaxis: chloroquine.

Grenada, Guadeloupe
Yellow fever vaccination certificate **required** from travellers over one year of age coming from infected areas.

Haiti
Yellow fever vaccination certificate required from travellers coming from infected areas.

Malaria risk (almost exclusively *P.falciparum*) throughout the year below 300m in suburban and rural areas.

Recommended prophylaxis: chloroquine.

Jamaica
Yellow fever vaccination certificate **required** from travellers over one year of age coming from infected areas.

Netherlands Antilles

Yellow fever vaccination certificate **required** from travellers over six months of age coming from infected areas.

Saint Kitts and Nevis, Saint Vincent and the Grenadines

Yellow fever vaccination certificate **required** from travellers over one year of age coming from infected areas.

Trinidad and Tobago

Yellow fever vaccination certificate required from travellers over one year of age coming from infected areas. Yellow fever vaccination usually advised for visits to rural or forested areas of Trinidad (not for solely city or beach holidays or for Tobago).

3.5   Tropical South America

(Bolivia, Brazil, Colombia, Ecuador including Galapagos, French Guiana, Guyana, Paraguay, Peru, Surinam, Venezuela including Marguerita island).

3.5.1   Disease risks

Food and water-borne diseases including amoebiasis, diarrhoeal diseases, helminth infections and hepatitis A are common. Bolivia, Brazil, Ecuador, Peru and Venezuela have all reported cholera.

Malaria (*P. falciparum*, *P. malariae* and *P. vivax*) in all countries. The main area of risk is the huge Amazon basin, largely in Brazil but extending into the adjacent countries. The falciparum malaria in the Amazon basin is highly chloroquine resistant.

Other arthropod-borne diseases (see Chapter 7) are an important cause of ill health:

- Jungle yellow fever in forest areas in all countries except Paraguay, areas west of the Andes, and the north eastern and southern states of Brazil.
- American trypanosomiasis (Chagas' disease) in most countries.
- Cutaneous and mucocutaneous leishmaniasis in all countries (the latter increasing in Brazil and Paraguay).
- Visceral leishmaniasis especially NE Brazil; less frequently in Colombia and Venezuela; rare in Bolivia and Paraguay; not known in Peru.
- Epidemics of viral encephalitis and dengue fever in some countries
- Bancroftian lymphatic filariasis is endemic in parts of Brazil, Guyana and Surinam.
- Onchocerciasis in isolated foci in rural areas of Ecuador, Venezuela and N Brazil.
- Bartonellosis or Oroya fever (sandfly-borne disease) on arid Western slopes of the Andes (up to 3,000m).
- Louse-borne typhus in mountain areas of Colombia and Peru.
- Myiasis
- Plague – some foci in Bolivia, Brazil, Ecuador and Peru.
- Relapsing fever.
- Rocky Mountain spotted fever in Colombia.

Diseases of close association:

- In 1994, an international commission certified the eradication of endemic wild poliovirus from the Americas. Ongoing surveillance in formerly endemic Central and South American countries confirms that poliovirus transmission remains interrupted.
- Meningococcal meningitis has occurred in epidemic outbreaks in Brazil.
- Tuberculosis endemic; incidence particularly high in Bolivia and Peru.

Sexually transmitted and blood-borne infections:
Hepatitis B of intermediate or high prevalence; highly endemic in the Amazon basin; HIV endemic.

Other hazards could include:
- Schistosomiasis in Brazil, Surinam and north-central Venezuela
- Rabies, snakes, leeches, dangerous fish and venomous spiders.
- Rodent-borne hantavirus infection and leptospirosis.

3.5.2 Recommendations for immunisations and malaria chemoprophylaxis (see later chapters for general health precautions)

FOR ALL COUNTRIES

Check routine immunisations including tetanus.

Immunisation against hepatitis A and typhoid recommended. Immunisation against yellow fever recommended for all countries except Paraguay but see details under individual countries.

For longer stays, consider immunisation against diphtheria and hepatitis B and check BCG status; for longer rural travel out of reach of medical attention consider immunisation against rabies.

3.5.3 Country by country variations and malaria chemoprophylaxis:

Bolivia
Yellow fever vaccination certificate required from travellers coming from infected areas. Recommended for incoming travellers from non-infected zones visiting risk areas such as the Departments of Beni, Cochabamba, Santa Cruz, and the sub tropical part of La Paz Department.

Malaria risk (predominantly *P.vivax*) throughout the year below 2500m in rural areas in several departments. Falciparum malaria occurs in the northern departments bordering Brazil. *P.falciparum* resistant to chloroquine and sulfadoxine-pyrimethamine reported.

Recommended prophylaxis: for rural areas below 2500m, chloroquine plus proguanil. In the northern borders near to Brazil, mefloquine (or doxycycline or atovaquone/proguanil) is more appropriate, as elsewhere in the Amazon basin.

Brazil
Yellow fever vaccination certificate **required** from travellers over nine months of

age coming from infected areas, unless they are in possession of a waiver stating that immunisation is contraindicated on medical grounds. The following countries or areas are regarded as infected:

- *Africa:* Angola, Cameroon, Democratic Republic of Congo, Gabon, Gambia, Ghana, Guinea, Liberia, Mali, Nigeria, Sierra Leone, Sudan.
- *America:* Bolivia, Colombia, Ecuador, Peru.

Vaccination is **recommended** for travellers to endemic areas including rural areas in Acre, Amapa, Amazonas, Goias, Maranhao, Mato Grosso, Mato Grosso do Sul, Pará, and Rondônia, Roraima and Tocantins, and certain areas of Minas Gerais, Parana and Sao Paulo. At present this does not include the tourist areas of Brazilia, Rio, Sao Paulo and Recife, unless outbreaks should occur.

Meningococcal A&C vaccine: consider for those living or working with local people.

Malaria risk throughout the year below 900m in the states of the legal Amazon region, including parts of the cities of Manaus and Porto Velho. *P.falciparum* highly resistant to chloroquine and resistant to sulfadoxine-pyrimethamine reported.

Recommended prophylaxis: in the 'legal Amazon', mefloquine (or doxycycline or atovaquone/proguanil); alternative chloroquine plus proguanil. Along the eastern seaboard and the arid areas inland from there, no antimalarials needed but travellers should be aware of the small risk.

Colombia

Immunisation against yellow fever **recommended** for travellers who may travel outside the capital and especially for the following areas: middle valley of the Magdalena river, eastern and western foothills of the Cordillera Oriental from the frontier with Ecuador to that with Venezuela, Uraba, foothills of the Sierra Nevada, eastern plains (Orinoquia) and Amazonia.

Malaria risk, predominantly *P.falciparum*, throughout the year in many rural areas below 800m of the following regions: Uraba (Antioquia and Choco Dep.), Bajo Cauca-Nechi (Antioquia and Cordoba Dep.), middle valley of the Magdalena river, Catatumbo (Norte de Santander Dep), whole Pacific Coast area, eastern plains (Orinoquia) and Amazonia. *P.falciparum* highly resistant to chloroquine and resistant to sulfadoxine-pyrimethamine reported.

Recommended prophylaxis: for most areas below 800m, chloroquine plus proguanil; in Amazonia, Pacifico and Uraba, mefloquine (or doxycycline or atovaquone/ proguanil).

Ecuador (including Galapagos)

Yellow fever vaccination certificate required from travellers over one year of age coming from infected areas, and recommended for all travellers to the low lands excluding Galapagos.

Malaria risk, roughly half *P.falciparum*, throughout the year below 1,500m in several provinces. No risk in Guayaquil or Quito. Chloroquine resistant *P.falciparum* reported. No malaria in Galapagos.

Recommended prophylaxis: chloroquine plus proguanil. In Esmeraldas province mefloquine (or doxycycline or atovaquone/proguanil) preferable.

French Guiana

Yellow fever vaccination certificate **required** from all travellers over one year of age.

Malaria risk, predominantly *P.falciparum*, throughout the year in the whole country. Resistance to chloroquine reported.

Recommended prophylaxis: mefloquine (or doxycycline or atovaquone/proguanil); alternative, chloroquine plus proguanil.

Guyana

Yellow fever vaccination certificate **required** from travellers coming from infected areas and from the following countries:

- *Africa:* Angola, Benin, Burkina Faso, Burundi, Cameroon, Central African Republic, Chad, Congo, Democratic Republic of Congo, Gabon, Gambia, Ghana, Guinea, Guinea-Bissau, Ivory Coast, Kenya, Liberia, Mali, Niger, Nigeria, Rwanda, Sao Tome and Principe, Senegal, Sierra Leone, Somalia, Tanzania, Togo, Uganda.
- *America:* Belize, Bolivia, Brazil, Colombia, Costa Rica, Ecuador, French Guiana, Guatemala, Honduras, Nicaragua, Panama, Peru, Surinam, Venezuela.

Yellow fever immunisation **recommended** for all travellers.

Malaria risk high throughout the year and in all interior regions including the north-west Region and areas along the Pomeroon river. Predominantly chloroquine resistant *P.falciparum*. Occasional cases in coastal belt.

Recommended prophylaxis: mefloquine (or doxycycline or atovaquone/proguanil); alternative chloroquine plus proguanil.

Paraguay

Yellow fever vaccination certificate **required** from travellers **leaving** Paraguay to go to endemic areas and from travellers arriving from endemic areas.

Malaria risk, largely *P.vivax*, in the Departments of Alto Paraná, Caaguazú, Canendiyú.

Recommended prophylaxis: for these areas only, chloroquine.

Peru

Yellow fever vaccination certificate **required** from travellers over six months of age coming from infected areas and **recommended** for those intending to visit areas of the country below 2,300m. Not for Lima, Machu Picchu and Cusco, including Lake Titicaca.

Malaria risk, predominantly *P.vivax*, throughout the year in almost all rural areas below 1,500m with chloroquine resistant falciparum malaria predominant in the Amazon basin. *P.falciparum* resistant to sulfadoxine-pyrimethamine also reported.

Recommended prophylaxis: for rural areas below 1,500m, chloroquine plus proguanil; mefloquine (or doxycycline or atovaquone/proguanil) in Amazon basin and swampy area west of the Andes bordering Ecuador.

Surinam
Yellow fever vaccination certificate **required** from travellers coming from infected areas and **recommended** for all travellers.

Malaria risk, predominantly *P.falciparum*, throughout the year in the three southern districts of the country; risk low in Paramaribo City and other coastal areas. Chloroquine resistant *P.falciparum* reported.

Recommended prophylaxis: for risk areas, mefloquine (or doxycycline or atovaquone/proguanil); alternative chloroquine plus proguanil.

Venezuela (including Marguerita Island)
Immunisation against yellow fever **recommended** for all travellers.

Malaria risk: *P.vivax* malaria widespread throughout the year in rural areas of: Amazonas, Apure, Barinas, Bolivar, Sucre and Tachira States. Caracas is free of malaria. Falciparum malaria in jungle areas of several provinces. Highly chloroquine resistant *P.falciparum* reported.

Recommended prophylaxis: chloroquine plus proguanil. None for Caracas, coastal areas or Marguerita Island. Mefloquine (or doxycycline or atovaquone/proguanil) is preferable for the Amazon basin area.

3.6 Temperate South America

(Argentina, Chile, Falkland Islands, Uruguay)

3.6.1 Disease risks

Food and water-borne diseases:
Gastrointestinal infections a risk in rural areas. Gastroenteritis (mainly salmonellosis) relatively common in Argentina, especially suburban areas. Hepatitis A and intestinal parasites reported.

Malaria confined to outbreaks in a few areas of NW Argentina.

Other arthropod-borne diseases (see Chapter 7) relatively unimportant except for American trypanosomiasis (Chagas' disease)
● Cutaneous leishmaniasis in NE Argentina.

Diseases of close association:
● In 1994, an international commission certified the eradication of endemic wild poliovirus from the Americas. Ongoing surveillance in formerly endemic Central and South American countries confirms that poliovirus transmission remains interrupted.
● Meningococcal meningitis outbreaks have occurred in Chile.
● Tuberculosis rates slightly higher than western Europe.

Sexually transmitted and blood-borne infections:
Hepatitis B of low prevalence; HIV generally of low prevalence.

Other hazards could include:
● Animal rabies endemic.
● Rodent-borne hantavirus pulmonary syndrome identified in north-central and SW regions of Argentina and in Chile.

3.6.2 Recommendations for immunisations and malaria chemoprophylaxis (see later chapters for general health precautions)

Check routine immunisations including tetanus.

For all countries *except the Falklands, immunisation against hepatitis A. Typhoid immunisation sometimes advised for rural backpackers.*

For longer travel, consider immunisation against diphtheria and hepatitis B and check BCG status; consider immunisation against rabies for longer rural travel out of reach of medical attention.

3.6.3 Country by country variations and malaria chemoprophylaxis:

Argentina

Malaria risk, exclusively *P.vivax*, confined to the north west area along the borders with Bolivia and Paraguay. The Iguassu Falls area is considered malaria free.

Recommended prophylaxis: for this small area in the NW corner of the country, which will rarely be visited by UK travellers, chloroquine.

3.7 North Africa and the Middle East, including Afghanistan and Turkey

(Afghanistan, Algeria, Bahrain, Egypt, Iran, Iraq, Israel, Jordan, Kuwait, Lebanon, Libya, Morocco, Oman, Qatar, Saudi Arabia, Syria, Tunisia, Turkey, United Arab Emirates, Yemen)

3.7.1 Disease risks

Food and water-borne diseases: particularly the dysenteries and other diarrhoeal diseases, hepatitis A, intestinal helminth infections including taeniasis (tapeworm), brucellosis and giardiasis. Typhoid fever and hepatitis E in some areas. Sporadic cases of cholera. Dracunculiasis in isolated foci in Yemen.

Malaria: limited but variable risk, especially towards the east and south of the area; see country by country guide below.

Other arthropod-borne diseases (see Chapter 7) generally not a major problem:
- Murine (endemic) and tick-borne typhus.
- Cutaneous leishmaniasis.
- Visceral leishmaniasis – central Iraq, SW Saudi Arabia, NW Syria, Turkey (SE Anatolia only) and Yemen.
- Relapsing fever.
- Rift Valley fever.
- Sandfly fever.
- West Nile fever in some areas.
- Crimean-Congo haemorrhagic fever in Iraq.
- Onchocerciasis – limited foci in Yemen.
- Filariasis – locally in the Nile delta.
- Plague foci.

Diseases of close association:
- Poliomyelitis – countries reporting polio cases in 1998 and 1999 include: Afghanistan, Egypt, Iraq, Turkey, Syria and Yemen.
- Tuberculosis endemic – most countries have incidence rates higher than in western Europe, particularly Afghanistan, Iraq, Morocco and Yemen.
- Trachoma.
- Meningococcal infection for pilgrims to Saudi Arabia.

Sexually transmitted and blood-borne infections:
Hepatitis B of intermediate prevalence; reported rates of HIV infection low for most countries.

Other hazards could include:

- Schistosomiasis (bilharziasis) especially Nile delta and Nile valley, SW Iran, Iraq, Saudi Arabia, Syria and Yemen.
- Rabies, snakes and scorpions.
- Dehydration and heat exhaustion for pilgrims to Mecca and Medina if the Hajj coincides with the hot season.

3.7.2 Recommendations for immunisations and malaria chemoprophylaxis (see later chapters for general health precautions)

> **FOR ALL COUNTRIES**
>
> *Check routine immunisations including tetanus.*
>
> *Immunisation against poliomyelitis (see 1.8), hepatitis A and typhoid for most countries; however, it should be noted that typhoid and/or hepatitis A are less important for short stays in tourist or business hotels.*
>
> *For longer stays, consider immunisation against diphtheria and hepatitis B and check BCG status; consider immunisation against rabies for longer rural travel.*

3.7.3 Country by country variations and malaria chemoprophylaxis:

Afghanistan

Yellow fever vaccination certificate **required** from travellers coming from infected areas.

Malaria risk, predominantly *P.vivax*, May-November below 2,000m. Chloroquine resistant *P.falciparum* in the south of the country.

Recommended prophylaxis: chloroquine plus proguanil.

Algeria

Yellow fever vaccination certificate **required** from travellers over one year of age coming from infected areas.

Malaria risk limited to a small focus of *P.vivax* in Ihrir (Illizi Dept) which is not usually visited by tourists. (Anyone going to this area should be aware of the risk).

Recommended prophylaxis: none.

Egypt

Yellow fever vaccination certificate required from travellers over one year of age coming from infected areas. (Air passengers in transit coming from these countries or areas without a certificate will be detained in the precincts of the airport until they resume their journey). The following countries and areas are regarded as infected:

● *Africa:* Angola, Benin, Burkina Faso, Burundi, Cameroon, Central African Republic, Chad, Congo, Democratic Republic of Congo, Equatorial Guinea, Ethiopia, Gabon, Gambia, Ghana, Guinea, Guinea-Bissau, Ivory Coast, Kenya, Liberia, Mali, Niger, Nigeria, Rwanda, Sao Tome and Principe, Senegal, Sierra Leone, Somalia, Sudan (south of 15°N), Tanzania, Togo, Uganda, Zambia.

● *America:* Belize, Bolivia, Brazil, Colombia, Costa Rica, Ecuador, French Guiana, Guyana, Panama, Peru, Surinam, Trinidad and Tobago, Venezuela.

All arrivals from Sudan are required to possess either a vaccination certificate or a location certificate issued by a Sudanese official centre stating that they have not been in Sudan south of 15°N within the previous six days.

Malaria risk: limited risk (*P.vivax* and *P.falciparum*) June–October and confined to the El Faiyum area which is 50 miles SW of Cairo and rarely visited by tourists.

Recommended prophylaxis: for tourist areas including Nile cruises – none; for the risk area, June–October, chloroquine.

Iran

Malaria risk (*P.vivax*) in parts of the central, western and south-western regions during the summer months. *P.falciparum* from March to November more in the south east. In practice this means there is limited risk over much of the country, greater risk in the south and especially the south-east. Chloroquine resistant *P.falciparum* reported.

Recommended prophylaxis: for areas outside the main cities, March-November, chloroquine plus proguanil.

Iraq

Yellow fever vaccination certificate **required** from travellers coming from infected areas.

Malaria risk, exclusively *P.vivax*, from May to November in some areas in the north below 1,500m (Duhok, Erbil, Ninawa, Sulaimaniya and Ta'min provinces), and also in Basrah province.

Recommended prophylaxis: for these rural areas in the North and for Basrah, May–November, chloroquine.

Jordan

Yellow fever vaccination certificate **required** from travellers over one year of age coming from infected areas.

Lebanon
Yellow fever vaccination certificate **required** from travellers coming from infected areas.

Libya
Yellow fever vaccination certificate **required** from travellers coming from infected areas.

Morocco
Malaria risk: limited risk of *P.vivax* malaria May–October in some rural areas.

Recommended prophylaxis: none, but remember slight risk.

Oman
Yellow fever vaccination certificate **required** from travellers coming from infected areas.

Malaria risk: limited risk, including *P.falciparum*, in rural areas. No transmission in Muscat. Chloroquine resistance reported.

Recommended prophylaxis: for rural areas, chloroquine plus proguanil.

Saudi Arabia
Yellow fever vaccination certificate required from all travellers coming from countries any part of which is infected.

Vaccination requirements for pilgrims to Mecca (Hajj) for 2001:
- Yellow fever: all travellers arriving in Saudi Arabia from countries known to be infected with yellow fever (as shown in the WHO Weekly Epidemiological Record), must present a valid yellow fever vaccination certificate. In the absence of such a certificate an individual will be vaccinated upon arrival and placed under strict surveillance for six days from the day of vaccination or the last date of potential exposure to infection.
- Meningococcal infection: all visitors arriving for 'Umra' or pilgrimage or seasonal work are requested to produce a certificate of vaccination against meningococcal A infection, issued not more than three years and not less than ten days before arrival in Saudi Arabia (but see below).
- Those arriving from countries in the African meningitis belt will be checked at entry points to ensure they are vaccinated. Cases with suspected meningococcal infection will be isolated and contacts put under close supervision. Chemoprophylaxis will be administered to all visitors from these countries to lower the carriage rate among them.
Source: Ministry of Health, Saudi Arabia.
- **NB. The new conjugate meningococcal (MenC) vaccine, which protects only against**

C strains, and the polysaccharide A&C vaccine give insufficent protection. From 2001, the UK recommends quadrivalent ACWY meningococcal polysaccharide vaccine, which also protects against W135 strains, for protection of pilgrims travelling to Saudi Arabia (see also 8.4.4).

Malaria risk, predominantly P.falciparum, throughout the year in most of the Southern Region (except the high altitude areas of Asir Province) and in certain rural areas of the Western Region. Chloroquine resistance reported.

Recommended prophylaxis: for risk areas, chloroquine plus proguanil.

Syria
Yellow fever vaccination certificate **required** from travellers coming from infected areas.

Malaria risk, exclusively *P.vivax*, from May to October along northern border areas, and especially in the north-east.

Recommended prophylaxis: for northern border areas, May–October, chloroquine.

Tunisia
Yellow fever vaccination certificate required from travellers over one year of age coming from infected areas.

Turkey
Malaria – potential risk, exclusively *P.vivax*, March–November in the plain around Adana, Antalya (Side) and SE Anatolia.

Recommended prophylaxis: for most tourist areas, none; for tourist areas along the south coast east of, and including, Side, and for those going to inland SE Turkey from March to November, chloroquine prophylaxis is recommended.

United Arab Emirates
Malaria risk confined to foothill areas and valleys in the mountainous regions of the northern Emirates. Not considered a risk in Abu Dhabi or in the cities of Dubai, Sharjah, Ajman and Umm al Qaiwain.

Recommended prophylaxis: for the northern rural areas of the emirates other than Abu Dhabi, chloroquine plus proguanil.

Yemen
Yellow fever vaccination certificate **required** from travellers over one year of age coming from infected areas.

Malaria risk, predominantly *P.falciparum*, throughout the year but mainly September–February, except in Aden and the airport perimeter. Chloroquine resistance reported.

Recommended prophylaxis: chloroquine plus proguanil.

3.8 Sub-Saharan and Southern Africa

(Angola, Benin, Botswana, Burkina Faso, Burundi, Cameroon, Cape Verde, Central African Republic, Chad, Comoros, Congo, Democratic Republic of Congo (formerly Zaire), Djibouti, Equatorial Guinea, Eritrea, Ethiopia, Gabon, Gambia, Ghana, Guinea, Guinea-Bissau, Ivory Coast, Kenya, Lesotho, Liberia, Madagascar, Malawi, Mali, Mauritania, Mauritius, Mayotte, Mozambique, Namibia, Niger, Nigeria, Reunion, Rwanda, Saint Helena, Sao Tome and Principe, Senegal, Seychelles, Sierra Leone, Somalia, South Africa, Sudan, Swaziland, Tanzania (including Zanzibar), Togo, Uganda, Zaire (see Democratic Republic of Congo), Zambia, Zimbabwe)

3.8.1 Disease Risks

Food and water-borne diseases highly endemic – intestinal helminth infections, the dysenteries and other diarrhoeal diseases including giardiasis, typhoid fevers and hepatitis A and E are widespread. Amoebiasis in southern countries. Cholera in many countries in the area. Dracunculiasis occurs in isolated foci.

Malaria: high transmission rate of *P.falciparum* in most areas except for the southern tip of the continent. There is no transmission above 3,000m altitude, nor in the islands of Reunion and the Seychelles, Lesotho and St. Helena; there is a little vivax malaria in Mauritius. Malaria in sub-Saharan Africa is highly resistant to chloroquine and the risk to travellers is great. See recommendations for individual countries below.

Other arthropod-borne diseases (see Chapter 7) are a major cause of morbidity in the area:

- Yellow fever – outbreaks occur periodically in unvaccinated populations within the endemic zones (see map on inside back cover). See recommendations for individual countries below.
- Lymphatic filariasis and onchocerciasis widespread.
- Cutaneous and visceral leishmaniasis – particularly drier areas; visceral leishmaniasis is epidemic in eastern and southern Sudan.
- Human trypanosomiasis (sleeping sickness) – small isolated foci in all countries except Djibouti, Eritrea, Gambia, Mauritania, Niger, Somalia, the island countries of the Atlantic and Indian Oceans, Lesotho, Saint Helena, South Africa and Swaziland. Transmission rate is high in north-western Uganda and very high in Angola, Democratic Republic of Congo and Southern Sudan and there is significant risk of infection in travellers visiting or working in rural areas.
- Louse, flea and tick-borne typhus.
- Plague – natural foci reported from Angola, Kenya, Madagascar, Malawi,

Mozambique, Uganda, Tanzania, Zambia, Zaire and Zimbabwe and some areas of Southern Africa; not usually a risk for tourists.
- Dengue and many other viral infections transmitted by mosquitoes, ticks, sandflies etc, some presenting as severe haemorrhagic fevers, throughout the region.
- The virus reservoir for Lassa fever (the multimammate rat) exists in some rural areas of West Africa.
- Ebola and Marburg haemorrhagic fevers are present, but reported only infrequently.
- Relapsing fever
- Rift Valley fever.
- West Nile fever.

Diseases of close association:
- Poliomyelitis in most countries except Cape Verde, Comoros, Mauritius, Reunion and the Seychelles. Southern Africa is an emerging poliomyelitis free zone.
- Tuberculosis incidence considered high.
- Meningococcal meningitis – epidemics occur throughout tropical Africa particularly in the savanna in the dry season, which varies from country to country and can be unpredictable.
- Trachoma.

Sexually transmitted and blood-borne infections:
Hepatitis B and HIV infection of high prevalence.

Other hazards could include:
- Tetanus common.
- Schistosomiasis throughout the area except Cape Verde, Comoros, Djibouti, Reunion and the Seychelles, Lesotho, Saint Helena.
- Rabies.
- Snake bites.
- Large animal attacks.

3.8.2 Recommendations for immunisations and malaria chemoprophylaxis (see later chapters for general health precautions)

FOR ALL COUNTRIES

Check routine immunisations including tetanus.

Immunisation against poliomyelitis, hepatitis A and typhoid.

Yellow fever immunisation for many countries – risk to the traveller varies with itinerary but immunisation is always advised within the endemic zone (unless travel is exclusively to urban areas at high altitude) and may be mandatory – see individual entries below.

Meningococcal A&C immunisation recommended for longer visits to certain countries (see entries below) especially if backpacking or living or working with local people, or if current outbreaks reported. The risk is greatest in the dry season, but these may vary within a country and from year to year. As a guide, dry season in West Africa is usually between November–May/June. In East Africa, seasons are variable.

For those on longer visits consider immunisation against diphtheria and hepatitis B and check BCG status; for rural visits out of reach of medical attention, consider immunisation against rabies.

Malaria prophylaxis: see individual countries. Unless otherwise indicated, the recommended prophylaxis for Sub-Saharan Africa is mefloquine or doxycycline or atovaquone/proguanil (malarone). For those such as some children and pregnant women unable to take any of these: chloroquine plus proguanil, remembering that this regimen is likely to be less protective than the first-choice recommendations.

3.8.3 Country by country variations and malaria chemoprophylaxis:

Angola

Yellow fever vaccination certificate required from travellers over one year of age coming from infected areas and recommended for all travellers.

Meningococcal A&C vaccine in certain circumstances (see recommendations for all countries above).

Malaria risk high in all areas throughout the year. Predominantly *P.falciparum*. *P.falciparum* resistant to chloroquine and sulphadoxine-pyrimethamine reported.

Recommended prophylaxis: see 3.8.2 above.

Benin

Yellow fever vaccination certificate **required** from **all** travellers over one year of age.

Meningococcal A&C vaccine in certain circumstances (see recommendations for all countries (3.8.2) above).

Malaria risk high in all areas throughout the year. Predominantly *P.falciparum*. Chloroquine resistant *P.falciparum* reported.

Recommended prophylaxis: see 3.8.2 above.

Botswana

Malaria risk, predominantly *P.falciparum*, from November to May/June in northern parts of the country: Boteti, Chobe, Ngamiland, Okavango and Tutume districts/subdistricts. Chloroquine resistant *P.falciparum* reported.

Recommended prophylaxis: for the northern half of the country from November to June, chloroquine plus proguanil.

Burkino Faso

Yellow fever vaccination certificate **required** from **all** travellers over one year of age.

Meningococcal A&C vaccine in certain circumstances (see recommendations for all countries (3.8.2) above).

Malaria risk high in all areas throughout the year. Predominantly *P.falciparum*. Chloroquine resistant *P.falciparum* reported.

Recommended prophylaxis: see 3.8.2 above.

Burundi

Yellow fever vaccination certificate **required** from travellers over one year of age coming from infected areas, and **recommended** for all travellers.

Meningococcal A&C vaccine in certain circumstances (see recommendations for all countries (3.8.2) above).

Malaria risk high in all areas throughout the year. Predominantly *P.falciparum*. Chloroquine resistant *P.falciparum* reported.

Recommended prophylaxis: see 3.8.2 above.

Cameroon

Yellow fever vaccination certificate **required** from **all** travellers over one year of age.

Meningococcal A&C vaccine recommended for northern region in certain circumstances (see recommendations for all countries (3.8.2) above).

Malaria risk very high in all areas throughout the year. Predominantly *P.falciparum*. *P.falciparum* resistant to chloroquine and sulphadoxine-pyrimethamine reported.

Recommended prophylaxis: see 3.8.2 above.

Cape Verde

Yellow fever vaccination certificate **required** from travellers over one year of age coming from countries having notified cases in the last six years; **recommended** for all travellers.

Malaria prophylaxis: none. Limited risk in Sao Tiago Island, no prophylaxis recommended but remember slight risk if fever occurs.

Central African Republic

Yellow fever vaccination certificate **required** from **all** travellers over one year of age.

Meningococcal A&C vaccine recommended for northern part in certain circumstances (see recommendations for all countries (3.8.2) above).

Malaria risk high in all areas throughout the year. Predominantly *P.falciparum*. Chloroquine resistant *P.falciparum* reported.

Recommended prophylaxis: see 3.8.2 above.

Chad

Yellow fever vaccination certificate recommended for all travellers over one year of age (yellow fever is endemic South of 15°N).

Meningococcal A&C vaccine recommended for southern part in certain circumstances (see recommendations for all countries (3.8.2) above).

Malaria risk high in all areas throughout the year. Predominantly *P.falciparum*. Chloroquine resistant *P.falciparum* reported.

Recommended prophylaxis: see 3.8.2 above.

Comoros

Malaria risk high in all areas throughout the year. Predominantly *P.falciparum*. Chloroquine resistant *P.falciparum* reported.

Recommended prophylaxis: see 3.8.2 above.

Congo

Yellow fever vaccination certificate **required** from **all** travellers over one year of age.

Malaria risk high in all areas throughout the year. Predominantly *P.falciparum*. Chloroquine resistant *P.falciparum* reported.

Recommended prophylaxis: see 3.8.2 above.

Democratic Republic of Congo (formerly Zaire)

Yellow fever vaccination certificate **required** from travellers over one year of age.

Malaria risk high in all areas throughout the year. Predominantly *P.falciparum*. Highly chloroquine resistant *P.falciparum* reported.

Recommended prophylaxis: see 3.8.2 above.

Djibouti
Yellow fever vaccination certificate **required** from travellers over one year of age coming from infected areas and **recommended** for all travellers.

Meningococcal A&C vaccine in certain circumstances (see recommendations for all countries (3.8.2) above).

Malaria risk high in all areas throughout the year. Predominantly *P.falciparum*. Chloroquine resistant *P.falciparum* reported.

Recommended prophylaxis: see 3.8.2 above.

Equatorial Guinea
Yellow fever vaccination certificate **required** from travellers coming from infected areas and **recommended** for all travellers.

Malaria risk high in all areas throughout the year. Predominantly *P.falciparum*. Chloroquine resistant *P.falciparum* reported.

Recommended prophylaxis: see 3.8.2 above.

Eritrea
Yellow fever vaccination certificate **required** from travellers coming from infected areas.

Meningococcal A&C vaccine in certain circumstances (see recommendations for all countries (3.8.2) above).

Malaria risk in all areas under 2,000m throughout the year. Asmara no risk. Predominantly *P.falciparum*.

Recommended prophylaxis: see 3.8.2 above

Ethiopia
Yellow fever vaccination certificate required from travellers over one year of age coming from infected areas and recommended for all travellers.

Meningococcal A&C vaccine recommended in certain circumstances (see recommendations for all countries (3.8.2) above).

Malaria risk, predominantly *P.falciparum*, in all areas under 2,000m throughout the year. Highly chloroquine resistant *P.falciparum* reported. No risk in Addis Ababa.

Recommended prophylaxis: see 3.8.2 above.

Gabon

Yellow fever vaccination certificate **required** from **all** travellers over one year of age.

Malaria risk high in all areas throughout the year. Predominantly *P.falciparum*. Chloroquine resistant *P.falciparum* reported.

Recommended prophylaxis: see 3.8.2 above.

Gambia

Yellow fever vaccination certificate **required** from travellers over one year of age arriving from endemic or infected areas and **recommended** for all travellers.

Meningococcal A&C vaccine recommended in certain circumstances (see recommendations for all countries (3.8.2) above). Not routinely recommended for tourist visits unless outbreak reported.

Malaria risk high in all areas throughout the year. Predominantly *P.falciparum*. Chloroquine resistant *P.falciparum* reported.

Recommended prophylaxis: see 3.8.2 above.

Ghana

Yellow fever vaccination certificate **required** from **all** travellers.

Meningococcal A&C vaccine recommended for northern area in certain circumstances (see recommendations for all countries (3.8.2) above).

Malaria risk very high in all areas throughout the year. Predominantly *P.falciparum*. Chloroquine resistant *P.falciparum* reported.

Recommended prophylaxis: see 3.8.2 above.

Guinea

Yellow fever vaccination certificate **required** from travellers over one year of age coming from infected areas and **recommended** for all travellers.

Meningococcal A&C vaccine recommended in certain circumstances (see recommendations for all countries (3.8.2) above).

Malaria risk high in all areas throughout the year. Predominantly *P.falciparum*. Chloroquine resistant *P.falciparum* reported.

Recommended prophylaxis: see 3.8.2 above.

Guinea – Bissau

Yellow fever vaccination certificate **required** from travellers over one year of age coming from infected areas and from the following countries:

- *Africa:* Angola, Benin, Burkina Faso, Burundi, Cape Verde, Central African Republic,

Chad, Congo, Democratic Republic of Congo, Djibouti, Equatorial Guinea, Ethiopia, Gabon, Gambia, Ghana, Guinea, Ivory Coast, Kenya, Liberia, Madagascar, Mali, Mauritania, Mozambique, Niger, Nigeria, Rwanda, Sao Tome and Principe, Senegal, Sierra Leone, Somalia, Tanzania, Togo, Uganda, Zambia

America: Bolivia, Brazil, Colombia, Ecuador, French Guiana, Guyana, Panama, Peru, Surinam, Venezuela

and **recommended** for all travellers.

Meningococcal A&C vaccine recommended in certain circumstances (see recommendations for all countries (3.8.2) above).

Malaria risk very high in all areas throughout the year. Predominantly *P.falciparum.* Chloroquine resistant *P.falciparum* reported.

Recommended prophylaxis: see 3.8.2 above.

Ivory Coast

Yellow fever vaccination certificate **required** from **all** travellers over one year of age.

Meningococcal A&C vaccine recommended for northern areas in certain circumstances (see recommendations for all countries (3.8.2) above).

Malaria risk very high in all areas throughout the year. Predominantly *P.falciparum.* Chloroquine resistant *P.falciparum* reported.

Recommended prophylaxis: see 3.8.2 above.

Kenya

Yellow fever vaccination certificate **required** from travellers over one year of age coming from infected areas, and **recommended** for all travellers, except those who confine their visit to a few days in Nairobi city.

Meningococcal A&C vaccine recommended in certain circumstances (see recommendations for all countries (3.8.2) above). Not routinely recommended for tourist visits unless outbreak reported.

Malaria risk very high in most areas throughout the year. The only areas where there is normally little risk are the centre of Nairobi and the highlands (above 2,500m) of Central, Rift Valley, Eastern, Nyanza and Western provinces. Predominantly *P.falciparum. P.falciparum* highly resistant to chloroquine and resistant to sulfadoxine-pyrimethamine reported.

Recommended prophylaxis: see 3.8.2 above.

Lesotho

Yellow fever vaccination certificate **required** from travellers coming from infected areas.

No malaria risk.

Recommended prophylaxis: none.

Liberia

Yellow fever vaccination certificate **required** from **all** travellers over one year of age.

Malaria risk very high in all areas throughout the year. Predominantly *P.falciparum*. *P.falciparum* highly resistant to chloroquine and resistant to sulphadoxine-pyrimethamine reported.

Recommended prophylaxis: see 3.8.2 above

Madagascar

Yellow fever vaccination certificate **required** from travellers coming from, or having been in transit in, areas considered to be infected.

Malaria risk in all areas throughout the year, especially in coastal areas. Predominantly *P.falciparum*. Chloroquine resistant *P.falciparum* reported.

Recommended prophylaxis: see 3.8.2 above

Malawi

Yellow fever vaccination certificate **required** from travellers coming from infected areas.

Meningococcal A&C vaccine recommended in certain circumstances (see recommendations for all countries (3.8.2) above).

Malaria risk very high in all areas throughout the year. Predominantly *P.falciparum*. *P.falciparum* highly resistant to chloroquine and resistant to sulphadoxine-pyrimethamine reported.

Recommended prophylaxis: see 3.8.2 above

Mali

Yellow fever vaccination certificate **required** from **all** travellers over one year of age (yellow fever is endemic south of 15°N).

Meningococcal A&C vaccine recommended for southern areas in certain circumstances (see recommendations for all countries (3.8.2) above).

Malaria risk high in all areas throughout the year. Predominantly *P.falciparum*. Chloroquine resistant *P.falciparum* reported.

Recommended prophylaxis: see 3.8.2 above.

Mauritania

Yellow fever vaccination certificate **required** from all travellers over one year of age, *except* those arriving from a non-infected area and staying in Mauritania less than two weeks.

Malaria risk, predominantly *P.falciparum*, throughout the year in all areas except Dakhlet–Nouadhibou and Tiris–Zemour, in the north. Risk in the north confined to the rainy season (Jul–Oct).

Recommended prophylaxis: in risk areas, chloroquine plus proguanil.

Mauritius

Yellow fever vaccination certificate **required** from travellers over one year of age coming from infected areas, considered to be those listed as endemic zones.

Malaria risk, exclusively *P.vivax*, throughout the year in certain rural areas; not Rodrigues Island.

Recommended prophylaxis: for rural areas, chloroquine. For other areas, remember slight risk if fever occurs.

Mozambique

Yellow fever vaccination certificate **required** from travellers over one year of age coming from infected areas.

Meningococcal A&C vaccine recommended in certain circumstances (see recommendations for all countries (3.8.2) above).

Malaria risk high in all areas throughout the year. Predominantly *P.falciparum*. *P.falciparum* highly resistant to chloroquine and resistant to sulphadoxine-pyrimethamine reported.

Recommended prophylaxis: see 3.8.2 above.

Namibia

Yellow fever vaccination certificate **required** from travellers coming from, or transitting on unscheduled flights through, infected areas. Travellers on scheduled flights which have transitted through infected areas are exempt provided they remained at the scheduled airport or adjacent town. A certificate is not insisted on for children under one year, but such infants may be subject to surveillance. The countries, or parts of countries, included in the endemic zones in Africa and South America are regarded as infected.

Meningococcal A&C vaccine recommended for north of country in certain circumstances. Not routinely recommended for tourist visits unless outbreak reported (see recommendations for all countries (3.8.2) above).

Malaria risk, predominantly *P.falciparum*, in northern regions (approximately one third of the country) from November to June and along the Kavango and Kunene rivers (the northern border) throughout the year. Resistance to chloroquine reported.

Recommended prophylaxis: chloroquine plus proguanil for northern area November–June, year round in extreme north.

Niger
Yellow fever vaccination certificate **required** from **all** travellers over one year of age and recommended for travellers leaving Niger. (Yellow fever is endemic south of 15°N).

Meningococcal A&C vaccine recommended for southern area in certain circumstances (see recommendations for all countries (3.8.2) above).

Malaria risk high in all areas throughout the year. Predominantly *P.falciparum*. Chloroquine resistant *P.falciparum* reported.

Recommended prophylaxis: see 3.8.2 above.

Nigeria
Yellow fever vaccination certificate **required** from travellers over one year of age coming from infected areas, and **recommended** for all travellers

Meningococcal A&C vaccine recommended for visits to northern part of the country in certain circumstances (see recommendations for all countries (3.8.2) above).

Malaria risk very high throughout the year in the whole country. Predominantly *P.falciparum*. Chloroquine resistance reported.

Recommended prophylaxis: see 3.8.2 above.

Reunion
Yellow fever vaccination certificate **required** from travellers over one year of age coming from infected areas.

No malaria risk.

Recommended prophylaxis: none.

Rwanda
Yellow fever vaccination certificate **required** from **all** travellers over one year of age.

Meningococcal A&C vaccine recommended in certain circumstances (see recommendations for all countries (3.8.2) above).

Malaria risk high in all areas throughout the year. Predominantly *P.falciparum*. *P.falciparum* highly resistant to chloroquine and resistant to sulphadoxine-pyrimethamine reported.

Recommended prophylaxis: see 3.8.2 above.

Saint Helena
Yellow fever vaccination certificate **required** from travellers over one year of age coming from infected areas.

Sao Tome and Principe
Yellow fever vaccination certificate **required** from **all** travellers over one year of age.

Malaria risk, predominantly *P.falciparum*, in all areas throughout the year. Chloroquine resistant *P.falciparum* reported.

Recommended prophylaxis: see 3.8.2 above.

Senegal
Yellow fever vaccination certificate **required** from travellers coming from endemic areas and **recommended** for all travellers.

Meningococcal A&C vaccine recommended for southern part of the country in certain circumstances (see recommendations for all countries (3.8.2) above).

Malaria risk high in all areas throughout the year. Predominantly *P.falciparum*. Chloroquine resistance reported.

Recommended prophylaxis: see 3.8.2 above.

Seychelles
Yellow fever vaccination certificate **required** from travellers over one year of age coming from infected areas or who have passed through partly or wholly endemic areas within the preceding six days. The countries and areas in the endemic zones are considered as infected areas.

No malaria risk.

Recommended prophylaxis: none.

Sierra Leone
Yellow fever vaccination certificate **required** from travellers coming from infected areas, and **recommended** for all travellers.

Malaria risk very high in all areas throughout the year. Predominantly *P.falciparum*. Chloroquine resistance reported.

Recommended prophylaxis: see 3.8.2 above.

Somalia
Yellow fever vaccination certificate **required** from travellers coming from infected areas, and **recommended** for all travellers.

Meningococcal A&C vaccine recommended in certain circumstances (see recommendations for all countries (3.8.2) above).

Malaria risk high in all areas throughout the year. Predominantly *P.falciparum*. Chloroquine resistant *P.falciparum* reported.

Recommended prophylaxis: see 3.8.2 above.

South Africa

Yellow fever vaccination certificate **required** from travellers over one year of age coming from infected areas. The countries or parts of countries included in the endemic zone in Africa and the Americas are regarded as infected.

Malaria risk, predominantly *P.falciparum*, throughout the year in low altitude areas of the northern and eastern Transvaal and eastern Natal as far south as the Tugela river (sixty miles north of Durban). At times of heavy rainfall this area may get larger and transmission rates may increase. Resistance to chloroquine reported.

Recommended prophylaxis: for risk areas (which are in the north eastern part of the country and include Kruger National Park), see 3.8.2 above.

Sudan

Yellow fever vaccination certificate **required** from travellers over one year of age coming from infected areas. The countries and areas included in the endemic zone are considered as infected. A certificate may be required from travellers leaving Sudan. **Recommended** for all travellers (yellow fever is endemic south of 12°N).

Meningococcal A&C vaccine recommended in certain circumstances (see recommendations for all countries (3.8.2) above).

Malaria risk high in all areas throughout the year. Predominantly *P.falciparum*. Highly chloroquine resistant *P.falciparum* reported.

Risk on the Red Sea coast is very limited, and that in the north and beside Lake Nasser is limited.

Recommended prophylaxis: see 3.8.2 above

Swaziland

Yellow fever vaccination certificate **required** from travellers coming from infected areas.

Malaria risk, predominantly *P.falciparum*, throughout the year in all low veld areas (mainly Big Bend, Mhlume, Simunye and Tshaneni). These are in the eastern half of the country. Highly chloroquine resistant *P.falciparum* reported.

Recommended prophylaxis: see 3.8.2 above.

Tanzania (including Zanzibar)

Yellow fever vaccination certificate **required** from travellers over one year of age coming from infected areas, regarded as those listed as endemic zones, and **recommended** for all travellers.

Meningococcal A&C vaccine recommended in certain circumstances (see recommendations for all countries (3.8.2) above).

Malaria risk very high throughout the year in all areas under 1,800m. Predominantly *P.falciparum*. *P.falciparum* highly resistant to chloroquine and resistant to sulphadoxine-pyrimethamine reported.

Recommended prophylaxis: see 3.8.2 above.

Togo

Yellow fever vaccination certificate **required** from **all** travellers over one year of age (yellow fever is endemic south of 15°N).

Meningococcal A&C vaccine recommended in certain circumstances (see recommendations for all countries (3.8.2) above).

Malaria risk high in all areas throughout the year. Predominantly *P.falciparum*. Chloroquine resistant *P.falciparum* reported.

Recommended prophylaxis: see 3.8.2 above.

Uganda

Yellow fever vaccination certificate **required** from travellers over one year of age coming from endemic areas and **recommended** for all travellers.

Meningococcal A&C vaccine recommended in certain circumstances (see recommendations for all countries (3.8.2) above).

Malaria risk very high throughout the year in the whole country including the main towns and cities. Predominantly *P.falciparum*. Chloroquine resistance reported.

Recommended prophylaxis: see 3.8.2 above.

Zaire – see Democratic Republic of Congo

Zambia

The western area is within the yellow fever belt; vaccination **recommended** for all travellers.

Meningococcal A&C vaccine recommended in certain circumstances (see recommendations for all countries (3.8.2) above).

Malaria risk high in all areas throughout the year. Predominantly *P.falciparum*. Highly chloroquine resistant *P.falciparum* reported.

Recommended prophylaxis: see 3.8.2 above.

Zimbabwe
Yellow fever vaccination certificate **required** from travellers coming from infected areas.

Meningococcal A&C vaccine recommended (May–October) in certain circumstances (see recommendations for all countries (3.8.2) above). Not routinely recommended for tourist visits unless outbreak reported.

Malaria risk, predominantly *P.falciparum*, from November to June in areas below 1,200m and throughout the year in the Zambezi valley. In Harare and Bulawayo the risk is negligible. Resistance to chloroquine reported.

Recommended prophylaxis: for the Zambezi valley, see 3.8.2 above. For other infected areas, chloroquine plus proguanil.

3.9   Indian Subcontinent

(Bangladesh, Bhutan, India, Maldives, Nepal, Pakistan, Sri Lanka)

3.9.1   Disease Risks

Food and water-borne diseases including cholera and other watery diarrhoeas, the dysenteries, typhoid fever, giardia and helminth infections. Hepatitis A very common. Large outbreaks of hepatitis E can occur.

Malaria present in all countries, except virtually eradicated from the Maldives.

Other arthropod-borne diseases endemic (see Chapter 7):

- Filariasis – common in Bangladesh, India and SW coastal belt of Sri Lanka
- Sandfly fever - increasing.
- Visceral leishmaniasis - sharp increase in Bangladesh, India and Nepal; also present in north Pakistan (Baltistan).
- Cutaneous leishmaniasis – India (Rajasthan) and Pakistan.
- Dengue - epidemics in Bangladesh, India (haemorrhagic in East), Pakistan and Sri Lanka (also haemorrhagic form).
- Japanese encephalitis occurs in much of the subcontinent. The risk is highest during and just after the rainy season.
- Plague – some natural foci in the area.
- Tick-borne and louse-borne relapsing fever and scrub typhus reported from India.

Diseases of close association:
- Polio eradication activities are as yet incomplete. Polio should still be assumed to be a risk to travellers.
- Meningococcal meningitis – outbreaks have occurred in Nepal.
- Tuberculosis incidence high.
- Trachoma in India, Nepal and Pakistan.

Sexually transmitted and blood-borne infections:
Hepatitis B of intermediate prevalence; HIV becoming more widespread.

Other hazards could include:
- Snakes.
- Rabies.

3.9.2 Recommendations for immunisations and malaria chemoprophylaxis (see later chapters for general health precautions)

FOR ALL COUNTRIES

Check routine immunisations including tetanus.

Immunisation against poliomyelitis, hepatitis A and typhoid.

For longer term travellers, check BCG status, and consider immunisation against diphtheria, hepatitis B and rabies.

For rural travel, usually for more than one month, particularly during and just after the rainy seasons, consider immunisation against Japanese encephalitis (see individual countries for risk). The vaccine is not necessary for the majority of travellers to the Indian subcontinent.

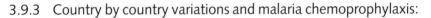

3.9.3 Country by country variations and malaria chemoprophylaxis:

Bangladesh

Yellow fever – any person (including infants) who arrives by air or sea without a yellow fever certificate is detained in isolation for a period of up to six days if arriving within six days of departure from an infected area or having been in transit in such an area, or having come by an aircraft that has been in an infected area and has not been disinsected in accordance with the procedure and formulation laid down in Schedule VI of the Bangladesh Aircraft (Public Health) Rules 1977 (First Amendment) or those recommended by WHO.

The following countries and areas are regarded as infected:
- *Africa:* Angola, Benin, Burkina Faso, Burundi, Cameroon, Central African Republic, Chad, Congo, Democratic Republic of Congo, Equatorial Guinea, Ethiopia, Gabon, Gambia, Ghana, Guinea, Guinea-Bissau, Ivory Coast, Kenya, Liberia, Malawi, Mali, Mauritania, Niger, Nigeria, Rwanda, Sao Tome and Principe, Senegal, Sierra Leone, Somalia, Sudan (south of 15°N), Tanzania, Togo, Uganda, Zambia.
- *America:* Belize, Bolivia, Brazil, Colombia, Costa Rica, Ecuador, French Guiana, Guatemala, Guyana, Honduras, Nicaragua, Panama, Peru, Surinam, Trinidad and Tobago, Venezuela.

Note: when a case of yellow fever is reported from any country, that country is regarded by the Government of Bangladesh as infected with yellow fever and is added to the above list.

Japanese encephalitis probably widespread but few data are available.

Malaria risk throughout the year in the whole country excluding Dhaka city. Risk highest along the northern and eastern borders and in the South East (Chittagong

Hill Tracts). *P.falciparum* highly resistant to chloroquine reported in the south-east and resistant to sulphadoxine-pyrimethamine reported from these latter areas.

Recommended prophylaxis: chloroquine plus proguanil; mefloquine (or doxycycline or atovaquone/proguanil) is appropriate for anyone visiting forested areas in the south east (including the Chittagong Hill Tracts).

Bhutan

Yellow fever vaccination certificate **required** from travellers coming from infected areas.

Meningococcal A&C vaccine recommended for all visits longer than a few days.

Japanese encephalitis may occur in the south, but few data are available.

Malaria risk throughout the year in the southern belt of five districts: Chirang, Gaylegphug, Samchi, Samdrupjongkhar and Shemgang. *P.falciparum* resistant to chloroquine and sulphadoxine-pyrimethamine reported.

Recommended prophylaxis: for risk areas in the southern districts, chloroquine plus proguanil.

India

Yellow fever – anyone (except infants up to the age of six months) arriving by air or sea without a yellow fever certificate is detained in isolation for up to six days if that person

(i) arrives within six days of departure from an infected area, or

(ii) has been in such an area in transit (excepting those passengers and members of crew who, while in transit through an airport situated in an infected area, remained within the airport premises during their entire stay and the Health Officer agrees to such exemption), or

(iii) has come on a ship that started from or touched at any port in a yellow fever infected area up to 30 days before its arrival in India, unless such a ship has been disinsected in accordance with the procedure laid down by WHO, or

(iv) has come by an aircraft which has been in an infected area and has not been disinsected in accordance with the provisions laid down in the Indian Aircraft Public Health Rules, 1954, or those recommended by WHO.

The following countries and areas are regarded as infected:

- *Africa:* Angola, Benin, Burkina Faso, Burundi, Cameroon, Central African Republic, Chad, Congo, Democratic Republic of Congo, Equatorial Guinea, Ethiopia, Gabon, Gambia, Ghana, Guinea, Guinea-Bissau, Ivory Coast, Kenya, Liberia, Mali, Niger, Nigeria, Rwanda, Sao Tome and Principe, Senegal, Sierra Leone, Somalia, Sudan, Tanzania, Togo, Uganda, Zambia.
- *America:* Bolivia, Brazil, Colombia, Ecuador, French Guiana, Guyana, Panama, Peru, Surinam, Trinidad and Tobago, Venezuela.

Note: when a case of yellow fever is reported from any country, that country is regarded by the Government of India as infected with yellow fever and is added to the above list.

Japanese encephalitis risk highest in central and north east India in the summer and autumn and in parts of the rural south all year round (see recommendations for all countries above).

Malaria risk throughout the year in the whole country below 2,000m. Urban transmission occurs. No transmission in certain parts of the states of Himachal Pradesh, Jammu and Kashmir, and Sikkim. Predominantly *P.vivax*, but *P.falciparum* is also important and mixed infections often occur. Highly chloroquine resistant *P.falciparum* reported.

Recommended prophylaxis: chloroquine plus proguanil except in mountain areas.

Maldives
Yellow fever vaccination certificate **required** from travellers coming from infected areas.

Malaria prophylaxis: none – malaria eradicated.

Nepal
Yellow fever vaccination certificate **required** from travellers coming from infected areas.

Meningococcal A&C vaccine recommended for all visits longer than a few days.

Japanese encephalitis occurs in the lowlands only, usually July–December (see recommendations for all countries).

Malaria risk, predominantly *P.vivax*, throughout the year in rural areas of the Terai districts (incl. forested hills and forest areas) of Dhanukha, Mahotari, Sarlahi, Rautahat, Bara, Parsa, Rupendehi, Kapilvastu, and especially along the Indian border. These are the lowland and foothill areas towards the southern border of the country and include the Chitwan National Park. No risk in Kathmandu. Chloroquine resistant *P.falciparum* reported.

Recommended prophylaxis: in risk areas, chloroquine plus proguanil.

Pakistan
Yellow fever vaccination certificate **required** from travellers coming from any part of a country in which yellow fever is endemic; infants under six months of age are exempt if the mother's vaccination certificate shows that she was vaccinated before the birth of the child. The countries and areas included in the endemic zones are considered as infected areas.

Japanese encephalitis may occur in the central area and outside Karachi, but few data available.

Malaria risk throughout the year in the whole country below 2,000m. Chloroquine resistant *P.falciparum* reported.

Recommended prophylaxis: chloroquine plus proguanil.

Sri Lanka

Yellow fever vaccination certificate required from travellers over one year of age coming from infected areas.

Japanese encephalitis can occur in lowland areas, especially northern and central provinces, usually October–January, but possibly also May–June (see 3.9.2).

Malaria risk, predominantly *P.vivax*, throughout the year in the whole country excluding the districts of Colombo, Kalutara and Nuwara Eliya. Chloroquine resistant *P.falciparum* reported.

Recommended prophylaxis: chloroquine plus proguanil. None in Colombo and districts listed.

3.10 South East Asia and the Far East

(Borneo (see Indonesia and Malaysia), Brunei Darussalam, Burma (see Myanmar), Cambodia, China (including Tibet), East Timor, Hong Kong (see China), Indonesia (including Bali and southern Borneo), Japan, Korea, Laos, Macao (see China), Malaysia (Peninsular Malaysia and northern Borneo, including Sarawak and Sabah), Mongolia, Myanmar (formerly Burma), the Philippines, Singapore, Taiwan, Thailand, Tibet (see China), Vietnam)

3.10.1 Disease risks

Food and water-borne diseases including cholera and other watery diarrhoeas, amoebic and bacillary dysentery, typhoid fever and hepatitis A and E. Flukes and intestinal parasites common among the indigenous population.

Malaria endemicity varies greatly but multidrug resistant *P.falciparum* common and specialist advice about appropriate prophylaxis may be necessary. See individual countries below.

Other arthropod-borne diseases (see Chapter 7) are an important cause of morbidity:
- Japanese encephalitis – endemic in rural areas; occasional urban outbreaks have been reported.
- Dengue – urban and rural epidemics occur.
- Filariasis – rural parts of many countries.
- Visceral leishmaniasis – recent resurgence in China.
- Cutaneous leishmaniasis – recently reported from Xinjiang.
- Plague in Vietnam, Myanmar, Mongolia, Indonesia and China; not usually a risk to tourists.
- Louse-borne relapsing fever.
- Lyme disease in some temperate regions.
- Scrub typhus and tularaemia.

Diseases of close association:
- Poliomyelitis – Polio eradication activities have rapidly reduced polio transmission in parts of this area. Elimination of polio reported in Brunei, Japan, Korea and Singapore. Transmission interrupted in China and probably interrupted in Indonesia, Laos, Malaysia, Myanmar, Philippines and Thailand. Mongolia no longer reports cases. There remains a focus of polio transmission in the Mekong Delta area of Cambodia and South Vietnam.
- Meningococcal infection – outbreaks of meningitis have occurred in Mongolia.
- Tuberculosis – incidence generally high, with some exceptions (such as Japan).

Sexually transmitted and blood-borne infections:
Hepatitis B of high prevalence; HIV endemic and spreading.

Other hazards could include:
- Schistosomiasis (bilharziasis) endemic in southern Philippines, central Sulawesi (Indonesia) and central Chang Jiang (Yangtze) river basin in China; small foci in Mekong delta in Vietnam.
- Rabies, snake bites and leeches.

3.10.2 Recommendations for immunisations and malaria chemoprophylaxis (see later chapters for general health precautions)

FOR ALL COUNTRIES

Check routine immunisations including tetanus.

Immunisation against poliomyelitis, hepatitis A and typhoid, noting that typhoid and/or hepatitis A may be less important for short stays in business or tourist hotels.

For longer term travellers, check BCG status and consider immunisation against diphtheria, hepatitis B and, for longer rural travel, rabies.

Japanese encephalitis immunisation (for individual countries see below) for rural travel, usually over one month. Less risk in dry seasons. Not recommended for most travellers.

3.10.3 Country by country variations and malaria chemoprophylaxis:

Borneo – see Indonesia and Malaysia

Brunei Darussalam
Yellow fever vaccination certificate **required** from travellers over one year of age coming from infected areas or who have passed through partly or wholly endemic areas within the preceding six days. The countries and areas included in the endemic zones are considered infected areas.

Japanese encephalitis – rural areas only; assume year round transmission.

Malaria: may be slight risk in border areas.

Recommended prophylaxis: none.

Burma – see Myanmar

Cambodia

Yellow fever vaccination certificate **required** from travellers coming from infected areas.

Japanese encephalitis – consider immunisation for some situations (see 3.10.2 above). Transmission season likely to be May-October.

Malaria risk, predominantly *P.falciparum*, throughout the year in the whole country except Phnom Penh area and close to Tonle Sap. Malaria does occur in the tourist area of Angkor Wat. *P.falciparum* highly resistance to chloroquine and resistant to sulphadoxine-pyrimethamine reported. Resistance to mefloquine also reported from western provinces.

Recommended prophylaxis: mefloquine, or doxycycline or atovaquone/proguanil (see 6.5); but mefloquine not suitable for western border areas.

China (including Hong Kong and Macao Special Administrative Regions)

Yellow fever vaccination certificate **required** from travellers coming from infected areas.

Japanese encephalitis in central and southern China, April/May–October; for northern China, the season is shorter. Consider immunisation in certain situations (see 3.10.2 above).

Malaria risk, predominantly *P.vivax*, below 1,500m in Fujian, Guangdong, Guangxi, Guizhou, Hainan, Sichuan, Xingjjang (only along the valley of the Yili river), Xizang (only along the valley of the Zangbo river in the extreme south) and Yunnan. Very low risk in Anhui, Hubei, Hunan, Jiangsu, Jiangxi, Shandong, Changhai and Zhejiang. Where transmission exists it occurs: north of 33oN, from July to November; between 33°N and 25°N, from May to December; and south of 25°N, throughout the year. Multidrug-resistant *P.falciparum* present in Hainan and Yunnan.

Recommended prophylaxis: main tourist areas – none; rural risk areas, chloroquine, except for Hainan and Yunnan provinces where mefloquine or doxycycline or atovaquone/proguanil (see 6.5) are the preferred drugs.

East Timor

Malaria risk- predominatly P. *falciparum* throughout the year in the whole territory. *P.falciparum* resistant to chloroquine and sulphadoxine pyrimethamine reported.

Recommended prophylaxis: mefloquine or doxycycline or atovaquone/proguanil (see 6.5).

Hong Kong and Macao, Special Administrative Regions of China

Malaria – No risk considered to exist in urban and most rural areas of Hong Kong. No risk in Macao.

Recommended prophylaxis: none.

Indonesia (including Bali and central/southern Borneo)

Yellow fever vaccination certificate **required** from travellers coming from infected areas. The countries and areas included in the endemic zones are considered by Indonesia as infected areas.

Japanese encephalitis probably year round. Consider immunisation in certain situations (see 3.10.2).

Malaria risk throughout the year in the whole country except in Jakarta Municipality, big cities, and the main tourist resorts of Java and Bali. *P.falciparum* highly resistant to chloroquine and resistant to sulphadoxine-pyrimethamine reported. *P.vivax* resistant to chloroquine is also reported in Irian Jaya.

Recommended prophylaxis: for Jakarta, big cities and main resort areas of Java and Bali, none, but remember the slight risk; for other areas, chloroquine plus proguanil. Mefloquine preferred for Irian Jaya.

Japan

Japanese encephalitis immunisation only recommended for rural travel, June–September (or April–October for south (Okinawa)) (see 3.10.2 above).

Korea (Democratic People's Republic of Korea and Republic of Korea)

Japanese encephalitis – immunisation only recommended for rural travel, July–October. (See 3.10.2).

Malaria – limited risk (exclusively *P.vivax*) in northern Kyunggi Do province.

Recommended prophylaxis: none.

Laos

Yellow fever vaccination certificate **required** from travellers coming from infected areas.

Japanese encephalitis, presumed season May–October. Immunisation recommended in certain circumstances (see 3.10.2 above).

Malaria risk, predominantly *P.falciparum*, throughout the year in the whole country except Vientiane. Highly chloroquine resistant *P.falciparum* reported.

Recommended prophylaxis: mefloquine or doxycycline or atovaquone/proguanil.

Malaysia (Peninsular Malaysia, northern part of Borneo including Sarawak and Sabah)

Yellow fever vaccination certificate **required** from travellers over one year of age coming from infected areas. The countries and areas included in the endemic zones are considered as infected areas.

Japanese encephalitis – year round transmission. Consider immunisation in certain circumstances (see 3.10.2).

Malaria risk limited to small foci in deep hinterland. Urban and coastal areas free from malaria except in Sabah where risk (predominantly *P.falciparum*) throughout the year. *P.falciparum* highly resistant to chloroquine and resistant to sulphadoxine-pyrimethamine reported.

Recommended prophylaxis: Peninsular Malaysia and Sarawak – none except for deep forests where chloroquine and proguanil; Sabah – mefloquine; alternatives doxycycline or atovaquone/proguanil (see 6.5); for shorter stays chloroquine plus proguanil is an acceptable alternative, but this regimen provides less protection.

Mongolia
Meningococcal vaccine recommended for longer visits.

Myanmar (formerly Burma)
Yellow fever vaccination certificate **required** from travellers coming from infected areas. Nationals and residents of Myanmar are required to possess certificates of vaccination on their departure to an infected area.

Japanese encephalitis – presumed season May–October. Consider immunisation in certain circumstances (see 3.10.2).

Malaria risk, predominantly *P.falciparum*, below 1,000 m
a. throughout the year in Karen State;
b. from March to December in Chin, Kachin, Kayah, Mon, Rakhine, and Shan States, Pegu Div., and Hlegu, Hmawbi, and Taikkyi townships of Yangon (formerly Rangoon) Div.;
c. from April to December in rural areas of Tenasserim Div.;
d. from May to December in Irrawaddy Div. and the rural areas of Mandalay Div.;
e. from June to November in the rural areas of Magwe Div., and in Sagaing Div.

P.falciparum highly resistant to chloroquine and resistant to sulfadoxine-pyrimethamine reported. *P.vivax* resistant to chloroquine reported.

Recommended prophylaxis: chemoprophylaxis is needed throughout Myanmar. For most of the country, mefloquine or doxycycline or atovaquone/proguanil. Doxycycline or atovaquone/proguanil on the Thai border.

Philippines
Yellow fever vaccination certificate **required** from travellers over one year of age arriving within six days from infected areas.

Japanese encephalitis – probably year round. Consider immunisation in certain circumstances (see 3.10.2).

Malaria risk throughout the year in rural areas below 600m, except for the provinces of Bohol, Catanduanes, Cebu and metropolitan Manila. The risk is low in the provinces of Aklan, Biliran, Camiguin, Capiz, Guimaras, Iloilo, Leyte del sur, Northern Samar, and Sequijor. Negligable risk in urban areas and the plains. Chloroquine resistant *P.falciparum* reported.

Recommended prophylaxis: for rural areas other than the four areas listed above, chloroquine plus proguanil; for other areas none, but be aware of the risk.

Singapore
Yellow fever vaccination certificate **required** from travellers over one year of age coming from infected areas. Certificates of vaccination are required from travellers over one year of age who, within the preceding six days, have been in or have passed through any country partly or wholly endemic for yellow fever. The countries and areas included in the endemic zones are considered as infected areas.

No malaria risk.

Recommended prophylaxis: none.

Taiwan
Japanese encephalitis – rural areas only, April–October. Consider immunisation in certain circumstances (see 3.10.2).

No malaria risk.

Recommended prophylaxis: none.

Thailand
Yellow fever vaccination certificate **required** from travellers over one year of age coming from infected areas. The countries and areas included in the endemic zones are considered as infected areas.

Japanese encephalitis – highest risk May–October. Consider immunisation in certain circumstances (see 3.10.2).

Malaria – no risk in cities nor in the main tourist resorts (such as Bangkok, Chiangmai, Pattaya, Phuket, Samui). Elsewhere there is malaria risk throughout the year. The risk is very low in the central plain, greater in forested and hilly areas of the country, especially in the areas bordering Myanmar, Laos and Cambodia. *P.falciparum* is highly resistant to chloroquine and sulphadoxine-pyrimethamine, and at the Myanmar and Cambodian borders also shows resistance to mefloquine and quinine.

While the city of Chiangmai is malaria-free, tourists commonly visit forested areas near the Myanmar border where there is a risk if they are there for an evening or night; some tourist hotels in NW Thailand are also very close to the forest. However, the combination of limited risk and resistance to several antimalarials means that most tourists will be advised not to take chemoprophylaxis; they must be made aware of the risk and that they must urgently seek prompt diagnosis and treatment in the event of fever during or up to a year after their visit.

Recommended prophylaxis: Bangkok and main tourist areas, none. Day visits to forested areas, none but be aware of the risk. Longer stays in rural areas with forests, and in border areas with Laos, Myanmar or Cambodia, doxycycline or atovaquone/proguanil.

Vietnam

Yellow fever vaccination certificate **required** from travellers over one year of age coming from infected areas.

Japanese encephalitis – Hanoi city and rural areas, highest risk May–October (see recommendations for all countries (3.10.2)).

Malaria risk, predominantly *P.falciparum*, in the whole country except urban centres, the Red River Delta, and coastal plains north of Nha Trang. High-risk areas are the two southernmost provinces of the country, Ca Mau and Bac Lieu, and the highland areas below 1,500m south of 18°N. *P.falciparum* highly resistant to chloroquine and resistant to sulphadoxine-pyrimethamine reported.

Recommended prophylaxis: mefloquine or doxycycline or atovaquone/proguanil in the risk areas.

3.11 Pacific Islands

(American Samoa, Cook Islands, Easter Island, Fiji, French Polynesia (Tahiti), Guam, Kiribati, Marshall Islands, Micronesia (Federated States of), Nauru, New Caledonia, Niue, Palau, Papua New Guinea, Samoa, Solomon Islands, Tokelau, Tonga, Trust Territory of the Pacific Islands, Tuvalu, Vanuatu and the Wallis and Futuna Islands)

3.11.1 Disease risks

Food and water-borne diseases:
Diarrhoeal diseases, typhoid fever, helminth infections and hepatitis A. Biointoxication may occur from raw or cooked fish or shellfish.

Malaria – endemic in Papua New Guinea, the Solomon Islands, and Vanuatu. Not in fiji nor in islands to the north, to French Polynesia and Easter Island in the east and to New Caledonia in the south (ie present in Melanesia, but absent from Polynesia and Micronesia due to absence of the vector mosquito).

Other arthropod-borne diseases (see Chapter 7):
- Filariasis – widespread but variable prevalence
- Dengue and dengue haemorrhagic fever – epidemics can occur in most islands
- Japanese encephalitis reported in the past from some islands including Guam, Saipan and recently from Papua New Guinea.
- Ross River fever
- Scrub typhus, mainly Papua New Guinea.

Diseases of close association:
- Poliomyelitis – poliomyelitis cases have not been reported from any of these areas for more than five years.
- Tuberculosis – variable incidence throughout the region – higher in Papua New Guinea.

Sexually transmitted and blood-borne infections:
Hepatitis B of intermediate to high prevalence and HIV reported.

Other hazards could include:
For sea bathers, corals, jellyfish, poisonous fish and sea snakes.

3.11.2 Recommendations for immunisations and malaria chemoprophylaxis (see later chapters for general health precautions)

FOR ALL COUNTRIES

Check routine immunisations including tetanus.

Immunisation against poliomyelitis, hepatitis A and typhoid.

For long term travellers, consider immunisation against diphtheria and hepatitis B and check BCG status.

3.11.3 Country by country variations and malaria chemoprophylaxis:

Fiji
Yellow fever vaccination certificate **required** from travellers over one year of age entering Fiji within ten days of having stayed overnight or longer in infected areas.

French Polynesia (Tahiti)
Yellow fever vaccination certificate **required** from travellers over one year of age coming from infected areas.

Kiribati
Yellow fever vaccination certificate **required** from travellers over one year of age coming from infected areas.

Nauru
Yellow fever vaccination certificate **required** from travellers over one year of age coming from infected areas.

New Caledonia and dependencies
Yellow fever vaccination certificate **required** from travellers over one year old coming from infected areas.

Cholera – vaccination against cholera is not required. Travellers coming from an infected area are not given chemoprophylaxis, but are required to complete a form for use by the Health Service.

Niue
Yellow fever vaccination certificate **required** from travellers over one year old coming from an infected area.

Palau

Yellow fever vaccination certificate **required** from travellers over one year of age coming from infected areas or from countries in any part of which yellow fever is endemic.

Papua New Guinea

Yellow fever vaccination certificate **required** from travellers over one year of age coming from infected areas.

Malaria – high risk, predominantly *P.falciparum*, throughout the year in the whole country below 1,800m. *P.falciparum* highly resistant to chloroquine and resistant to sulphadoxine-pyrimethamine reported.

Recommended prophylaxis: mefloquine or doxycycline or atovaquone/proguanil, or if these contra-indicated, maloprim plus chloroquine.

Japanese encephalitis – probably year-round risk. Consider immunisation for visits over one month to rural areas.

Samoa

Yellow fever vaccination certificate required from travellers over one year old coming from infected areas.

Solomon Islands

Yellow fever vaccination certificate required from travellers coming from infected areas.

Malaria – high risk throughout the year except in some eastern and southern outlying islets. Chloroquine resistant *P.falciparum* reported.

Recommended prophylaxis: mefloquine or doxycycline or atovaquone/proguanil, or if these contra-indicated, maloprim plus chloroquine.

Tonga

Yellow fever vaccination certificate **required** from travellers over one year of age coming from infected areas.

Vanuatu

Malaria – low to moderate risk, predominantly *P.falciparum*, throughout the year in the whole country. *P.falciparum* highly resistant to chloroquine and resistant to sulphadoxine-pyrimethamine reported.

Recommended prophylaxis: mefloquine or doxycycline or atovaquone/proguanil, or if these contra-indicated, maloprim plus chloroquine.

Accidents, injuries and recreational water hazards 4

4.1 Introduction

Accidents and injuries are a major cause of serious health problems abroad. About one third of a series of over 7000 medical cases reported to insurers were due to accidents. Many of these were preventable. The sense of excitement which travel induces may mean that the normal checks and precautions of everyday life are ignored. This is even more likely if influenced by alcohol.

Some of the more important risks for travellers are outlined below.

4.2 Transport

Roads: Traffic driving on the right presents a hazard to both drivers and pedestrians. It is easy to forget the direction from which traffic will be coming. Those responsible for children should take particular care.

Motor vehicles may be poorly maintained; brakes and tyres may be defective.

Driving: Other drivers may not observe rules. Even if there are no safety belt laws or speed limits in the country visited, seatbelts should be worn and speed kept to a suitable maximum and never above 70 miles an hour. Travellers should not be tempted to drive a motor cycle or moped without a helmet and adequate insurance. Any local religious and cultural rules must be acknowledged eg avoidance of sacred cows in Hindu areas. Women are not allowed to drive in certain Muslim countries. It may be more sensible for visitors to use a local driver.

Airlines: Some are safer than others (published data are available).

Ferries: Passenger ships on the whole have a good safety record; ferries, particularly in developing countries, are often overcrowded and carry inadequate lifesaving devices.

Public transport: Trains and coaches may be overcrowded; local habits such as travelling on the roofs of trains, jumping off trams and jay walking are dangerous.

4.3 Accommodation

Hotels may be built to poor standards and have inadequate fire escapes. It is a sensible precaution to note the site of emergency exits. Balconies may be unsafe and gas and electrical appliances may be in a dangerous condition.

4.4   Going out

Although muggings and murders hit the headlines, minor injury from snatching handbags and briefcases is much more common. Travellers can be easy targets by being unfamiliar with the language and surroundings and carrying more money and equipment than locals. It is best to behave in a low key manner and blend into the background, not to carry all possessions but use the hotel safe, and, if attacked, not to fight. It is sometimes wise to carry a small amount of money separately to hand over to thieves.

Many areas are not safe to wander around at night, including some which look pleasant and easy-going by day.

In some countries, producing cameras, computers or tape-recorders at the wrong time (eg near airports, railway stations) can result in arrest on suspicion of spying.

4.5   Water hazards

The dangers of water include infection as well as injury.

4.5.1   Swimming

Half the deaths due to drowning occur within two metres of safety. Local knowledge is essential to avoid dangerous currents. Diving into water of unknown depth or hazard (eg rocks) is a common cause of severe injury. One of the most dangerous dives is the running dive through surf on a gently sloping sandy beach. Children must be supervised at all times by an adult who can swim well.

Cold water is particularly dangerous and the initial physiological responses to the temperature can cause even strong swimmers to drown.

4.5.2   Infection

Visibly dirty recreational water is likely to be infected and should be avoided; also, someone in difficulties on the bottom of a murky pool may not be easily seen. Seawater is to a large extent self-cleansing, but obviously risky sites such as sewerage outlets should be avoided.

All rivers, lakes and fresh water in the tropics and sub-tropics should be assumed to be colonised with snails infected with schistosomiasis (bilharzia). The River Nile, and in Africa, Lakes Kariba, Malawi, Tanganyika and Victoria, are all infected. Wading or swimming in slow flowing rivers or lakes within endemic areas should be discouraged.

Leptospirosis can also be contracted by direct contact with water (including recreational water) contaminated by animals such as small rodents. It occurs worldwide.

4.5.3 Bites

Water is the home of many dangerous animals including sharks, crocodiles and hippopotamuses, Moray and Conger eels, groupers and garfish. Fish may also electrocute (electric eels, electric catfish, torpedo rays) or sting (weeverfish, stonefish, stingrays, scorpion fish, jellyfish, octopus). Local knowledge may help to avoid these dangers. (See Chapter 12 for more detail).

4.6 Hazardous sports and water sports

Appropriate life jackets or buoyancy aids should always be worn for sailing and windsurfing and for other water-linked sports such as angling.

Pursuits such as scuba diving, mountain climbing and hang gliding can be dangerous in unfamiliar surroundings and are best learnt in the UK before going abroad. Additional insurance may be required to cover such activities and travellers should make their insurers aware of their intention to take part in any such activities. At least 24 hours should be allowed between a dive and a flight.

4.7 Alcohol and drugs

All risks are magnified by alcohol. The general advice not to drink and drive applies as much abroad as it does at home. It is easy to drink more in a hot climate, and local drinks may be stronger than expected. There may be an expectation that over indulgence in alcohol and in some circles, drugs, are an essential part of the holiday experience. Business travellers may find that local hospitality includes potent alcoholic drinks. The possession of illicit drugs carries very severe penalties in some countries.

4.8 Political unrest

Up to date information is available from the Foreign and Commonwealth Office on areas of political unrest or terrorism (see Appendix 2, FCO website – http://www.fco.gov.uk). Information from local residents may be unreliable.

4.9 Insurance

Some countries, but by no means all, have reciprocal health care arrangements with the UK or are fellow members of the European Economic Area. Details are in the Department of Health leaflet, *Health Advice for Travellers* (T6). In general, they provide emergency treatment to the same standards as the local population, which may be less than we expect through our NHS; they may not cover all costs and there is no provision for repatriation of the very ill, or of human remains. Travel insurance covering both injuries and illness while travelling is therefore essential. It must be adequate in financial terms for the country or countries visited, must cover the risks of the trip and must include adequate funds for repatriation. The insurance should also include a 24-hour assistance service.

Prevention of travellers' diarrhoea and other food and water-borne diseases

5

5.1   Introduction

Travellers' diarrhoea, typhoid fever, cholera and hepatitis A can all be acquired by ingesting contaminated food or water. Travellers' diarrhoea occurs in up to a half of European travellers who spend three weeks or more in the developing areas of Africa, Latin America, the Middle East or Asia, even if they stay in good quality hotels. It should therefore be taken seriously.

The commonest organism associated with travellers' diarroea in tropical and subtropical areas is enterotoxigenic Escherichia coli, which may be part of the normal bowel flora of the local population. However, a range of bacteria, viruses and parasites are associated with the condition, including campylobacter, salmonella, shigella, and, especially in children, rotavirus. The main parasitic cause is Giardia lamblia.

5.2   Prevention

Spread is by the faecal-oral route, usually via food or water. Travellers can reduce the risk of disease by observing the precautions listed under 5.4.

5.3   Management of travellers' diarrhoea

Travellers' diarrhoea is usually a mild disease, though severe fluid and electrolyte disturbance may occur. Treatment is to replace fluid loss with a suitable oral solution; in severe cases parenteral replacement therapy may be required.

Travellers should preferably go prepared with commercial sachets of replacement sugar and salt which can be made up with freshly boiled or bottled water when needed. An alternative is to dissolve one teaspoon of sugar and a pinch of salt in a glass or mug (about 250ml) of freshly boiled or bottled water, flavoured to taste with fresh orange juice.

The sufferer should continue to eat what he/she feels like – food shortens the illness and lessens fluid loss.

Antimotility drugs may give symptomatic relief but should not be given to children or if there is fever.

Medical help should be sought if any one or more of the following occur:

- there is blood in the faeces
- the illness is accompanied by fever
- the affected person becomes confused
- the diarrhoea does not settle within 72 hours (24 hours for small children and the elderly)

Antibiotic prophylaxis is only occasionally appropriate for travellers' diarrhoea for those in whom the effects of the illness would be serious. Alternatively, for these travellers, antibiotics may be carried for immediate self treatment until medical help can be obtained.

In travellers without intercurrent disease, self therapy with antibiotics (e.g. ciprofloxacin) is not routinely recommended, although it may shorten the symptoms. If such medication is being prescribed it should be understood by the traveller that travellers' diarrhoea is essentially a self limiting disease, and whilst treatment is usually successful and trouble free, it could produce side effects, complicate the diagnosis and encourage the development of antibiotic resistance. A shortened course of ciprofloxacin is usually effective and should minimise the above disadvantages, but it should be remembered that extensive use of ciprofloxacin will mean it rapidly becomes ineffective worldwide. Ciprofloxacin should not be prescribed for children.

5.4 Rules for eating and drinking safely

Travellers should be reminded of the precautions they can take to eat and drink safely:

Eat and drink safely

Always wash your hands after going to the lavatory, before handling food and before eating.

If you have any doubts about the water available for drinking, washing food or cleaning teeth, boil it, sterilise it with disinfecting tablets or use bottled water – preferably carbonated with gas – in sealed containers.

Avoid ice unless you are sure it is made from treated or chlorinated water. This includes ice used to keep food cool as well as ice in drinks.

It is usually safe to drink hot tea or coffee, wine, beer, carbonated water and soft drinks, and packaged or bottled fruit juices.

Food may be contaminated even though it looks, smells and tastes perfectly normal, so avoid:

- *salads*
- *uncooked fruit and vegetables, unless you can peel or shell them yourself*
- *food which has been kept warm*
- *food likely to have been exposed to flies*
- *dishes containing uncooked egg*
- *ice cream from unreliable sources, such as kiosks or itinerant traders*
- *shellfish, especially if uncooked*
- *unpasteurised dairy produce*
- *food from street traders unless you are sure it is freshly prepared and hot*

Eat freshly cooked food which is thoroughly cooked and still piping hot.

6 Prevention of malaria

6.1 Introduction

About 2,000 cases of imported malaria are reported each year in the UK. While this total has changed little in recent years, the proportion due to the more severe *Plasmodium falciparum* has steadily increased. About seven people die from malaria each year in the UK and almost all these deaths are preventable.

Most cases of malaria are in those who failed to take, or comply regularly with, malaria prophylaxis. At particular risk are settled migrants returning to visit relatives abroad: they are often unaware that any natural immunity gained during residence in an endemic area rapidly wanes on leaving it. Malaria transmission may also have increased since they left. Most deaths from malaria have followed a delay in diagnosis because neither the returned traveller nor the doctor took prompt medical action for illness and/or fever.

Many warm climate countries are endemic for malaria and thus pose some risk to travellers. The level of risk may vary enormously between, and even within, countries and this will affect the type of prophylaxis recommended. Appropriate chemoprophylaxis combined with prudent behaviour can greatly reduce the risk, but the possibility of acquiring malaria remains whatever precautions have been taken. In all malarious areas the traveller must be aware of this risk and suspect any illness with fever to be possible malaria. This means getting prompt medical attention and, if back in the UK, pointing out to the doctor the history of travel to a malarious area.

6.2 Principles of malaria prevention

Since no chemoprophylactic regimen can be considered 100 per cent effective, chemoprophylaxis is only part of malaria prevention, which has four main components:

A. **A**wareness of the risk, by traveller and doctor.
B. Reducing **B**ites from anopheline mosquitoes.
C. Using appropriate **C**hemoprophylactic drugs.
D. Awareness of the residual risk, and prompt **D**iagnosis and treatment of clinical malaria.

6.3 Awareness of the risk

Both traveller and doctor need to be aware of the malaria risk during the planned visit, to select appropriate preventive measures, and to ensure prompt medical attention, diagnosis and treatment if malaria occurs in spite of precautions. The first is to prevent malaria, the second to prevent a fatal outcome and shorten the illness.

Malaria risk is set out in the previous pages by geographical region and by country, and these should be consulted. The situation in broad terms is as follows:

Most of **Africa south of the Sahara** is highly malarious and the vast majority of cases of falciparum malaria reported in England and Wales are acquired in East, West or Central Africa. The highest attack rates – around one to two per cent of travellers per visit in one study – occur in West Africa (Gambia, Ghana, Nigeria, Sierra Leone); attack rates in East Africa (Kenya and Uganda) are lower but more people visit this area and Kenya has been a particular source of fatalities. Some cities, but by no means all, are malaria-free. Chloroquine resistance is widespread throughout the continent and *P.falciparum* resistant to several common antimalarials occurs at varying levels throughout Africa south of the Sahara.

In **southern Africa** the risk of malaria is on the whole low, and large areas of Namibia and Botswana, parts of Zimbabwe, and South Africa except for certain game parks and rural regions in the north-east, are malaria-free. The areas affected and transmission of malaria may increase in times of heavy rainfall.

Thirty per cent of malaria imported into Britain is from the **Indian subcontinent**, mainly due to *P.vivax*. Some chloroquine resistance is reported.

Many popular tourist destinations in **south east Asia** are malaria free or have a very low risk. UK tourists infrequently visit regions of high transmission. Multi-drug resistant falciparum malaria occurs in Vietnam, Cambodia and the Thai–Cambodian border, making drug prophylaxis difficult.

In the **Pacific**, Papua New Guinea, Irian Jaya, the Solomon Islands and Vanuatu are malarious, and chloroquine resistant *P.vivax* as well as *P.falciparum* malaria is now reported. This is a cause for concern for future prophylaxis advice.

Latin America is a relatively infrequent destination for British travellers. In the central American republics, *P.vivax* predominates and although the risk is low, prophylaxis is recommended. In South America the whole Amazon basin is malarious with *P.falciparum* resistant to chloroquine (and often also sulphadoxine-pyrimethamine) present. Outside that large area risk is low in Brazil and negligible in its cities.

Different types of travel carry different risks. The package tourist who stays in one place will usually have a clearly defined risk (often high in Africa, but low in Asia), but beware the person with an urban destination who may add on visits to the countryside or game parks. Business travellers may be visiting downtown offices only, but they may be concerned with field projects or add a touristic weekend.

Overland travellers are at particular risk, especially if young – they may be exposed to a variety of environments and are unlikely to stay in screened air-conditioned hotels. Prolonged travel increases the risk of contracting malaria and the temptation to relax compliance with preventive measures must be resisted. This also applies to expatriates intending to reside in malarious areas for years – they may benefit from specialist advice.

Certain individuals are at higher risk of severe malaria and need to be fore-warned. These include pregnant women (See 15.2), and asplenic individuals. Malaria in pregnancy is often a life-threatening infection and the wisdom of travelling to a malarious area should always be questioned.

6.4 Protection against mosquito bites

It is important to reduce the chance of an infective mosquito bite as far as possible. Anopheles mosquitoes bite only between dusk and dawn, and most intensively during the night. To avoid being bitten travellers should be advised to take the precautions mentioned below.

Protection against mosquito bites

In the evenings, *wear long-sleeved shirts and long trousers, protect exposed limbs with a diethyltoluamide-containing repellant and wear diethyltoluamide-soaked ankle and wrist bands.*

Diethyltoluamide (DEET) is the most effective repellent and there is vast experience of its use since 1957. It is estimated to be used by 200 million people each year. DEET products should be applied with care to the face as they can irritate mucosal membranes (a skin test can be tried in advance). Most diethyltoluamide preparations remain effective on the skin for only two to four hours and therefore need regular re-application. Extended duration formulations are desirable (when available).

Children require similar measures, although there have been rare reports of toxicity following excessive use of diethyltoluamide in young children.

Mosquitoes may bite through thin material. An insecticide spray (permethrine) has recently become available for spraying on to clothing and is expected to be effective for two weeks.

Sleep *in fully air-conditioned or screened accommodation. Rooms should also be sprayed with a knockdown insecticide each evening after sundown to eliminate mosquitoes which entered during the day.*

Where the room cannot be made safe from insects, use a permethrin-impregnated bed net. This provides much greater protection than an ordinary net. Kits for impregnating nets are available – a single treatment lasts several months. Use an electrical pyrethroid vaporiser overnight where nets are not used.

6.5 Chemoprophylaxis

UK chemoprophylaxis regimens should always be advised in conjunction with advice on personal protection and recognition of malaria symptoms. Weekly drug regimens should be started at least one week before departure (preferably two to three weeks for mefloquine) and continued compliantly until four weeks after return. The first part of this advice is so that side effects or reactions may occur before departure, and can be dealt with before travelling. The continued use of drugs on return will deal with infection contracted towards the end of the stay. Possible side effects should be discussed. Minor side effects are frequent with all regimens. Users should be warned to get further advice if they are concerned about side effects or they are too severe to continue the medication. The chemoprophylactic should be taken after meals.

Travellers should also be warned that if they buy antimalarials abroad, the strength of the tablets may be different; they may need to take expert advice about how many to take to avoid unwittingly under-dosing.

Specialist advice is needed on antimalarial drugs for those with severe hepatic or renal impairment.

Chloroquine
In the absence of chloroquine resistant parasites, the adult dose of chloroquine 300mg (as base) (two tablets) weekly gives good protection against malaria attacks safely and with few side effects. This will not prevent establishment of the dormant liver stages of vivax and ovale malaria which can occasionally give rise to late attacks of malaria up to a year after travel.

Chloroquine plus proguanil
In areas with moderate to high chloroquine resistance, such as in sub-Saharan Africa, this combination now provides substantially less protection than mefloquine. For areas with limited chloroquine resistance chloroquine plus proguanil is still widely recommended and still has important advantages over newer regimens. It has a wide safety margin with no severe or permanent toxicity and has been used for many years in pregnancy and in infants, with no record of fetal toxicity. Folate supplements are recommended during pregnancy. For adults, the recommended doses are chloroquine 300mg (as base) (two tablets) weekly and proguanil 200mg (two tablets) daily. Compliance with daily dosing may be poor. Adverse reactions include nausea, diarrhoea, dyspepsia and itching. Chloroquine, but not proguanil, is available as a syrup; crushing proguanil tablets, for example in jam or butter, remains an unsatisfactory method of administering it to infants and young children.

Mefloquine

For areas such as sub-Saharan Africa where highly chloroquine resistant falciparum malaria occurs, weekly mefloquine (adult dose 250 mg weekly) is an effective regimen, and can be recommended for journeys up to one year in length. In Africa and the Pacific its efficacy is estimated to be 90 per cent, however resistance is high in parts of Cambodia and in Thailand on the Myanmar and Cambodia borders. Its single weekly dose appeals to travellers. Despite much media attention to them, major adverse events (convulsions, coma and psychotic disturbances) are rare – reported in about one in every 10,000 users taking prophylactic doses. Lesser side effects occur with a frequency similar to side effects from chloroquine and proguanil. For mefloquine these lesser side effects include dizziness, strange dreams, mood swings, insomnia, headaches and diarrhoea. These could affect the ability to drive, pilot a plane or operate machinery. The drug is only slowly excreted.

Mefloquine should not be given to people with a history of psychiatric disturbance or epilepsy. Mefloquine is currently not routinely advised during pregnancy. Where a pregnant traveller cannot be dissuaded from visiting areas with a high risk of highly chloroquine resistant *P. falciparum* malaria, it can be used cautiously during the second and third trimesters; data so far suggest it is also safe in the first trimester. Mefloquine is secreted in breast milk and in view of limited data, the manufacturer does not recommend its use during breastfeeding.

Malarone

Malarone is a combination of proguanil and atovaquone. It has proved highly effective in clinical trials in Africa as a prophylactic against *P. falciparum* malaria, with an overall efficacy of 98 per cent. It has been licensed for treatment of malaria in many countries including the UK for some time. It is now licensed in the UK for malaria prophylaxis in adults for up to 28 days. The PHLS Malaria Advisory Committee considers it an alternative to mefloquine or doxycycline to be considered for adults traveling to chloroquine resistant areas, particularly in Africa and SE Asia. It is taken as a single daily tablet and as it appears to act against the pre-erythrocytic stages of *P. falciparum* it only needs to be continued for seven days post travel.

The combination seems to be well tolerated. Reported adverse events have been mainly gastrointestinal – abdominal pain, dyspepsia, gastritis, and diarrhoea – although headaches are also commonly reported.

Doxycycline

In recent years increasing use of doxycycline for malaria prophylaxis in UK travellers has revealed few problems, although the overall number of users has been relatively low, partly due to its previously unlicensed status as a prophylactic in the UK. Doxycycline is now licensed for malaria prophylaxis and experience in its use for this indication is likely to increase.

Doxycycline is recommended for travellers to areas where *P.falciparum* strains are resistant to other drugs eg sub-Saharan Africa, western provinces of Camdodia and on the Thai–Myanmar and Thai–Cambodian borders. It is also recommended as an equal alternative to mefloquine for those areas of the Pacific Islands where malaria is endemic. In addition it is available as a second line regimen where mefloquine or chloroquine are unsuitable.

For travel to most areas of sub-Saharan Africa chloroquine plus proguanil has been the traditional alternative regimen, however doxycycline is considered, on the basis of trials outside Africa, to give greater protection than this combination. Those who are travelling to Africa for whom high levels of protection against malaria are desirable, but for whom mefloquine is unsuitable, may be recommended to use doxycycline.

Its main side effects are diarrhoea (but it can also provide protection against bacterial diarrhoeas), vaginal thrush and photosensitive dermatitis. The latter may be particularly relevant to those on beach holidays. It is not recommended for children under 12 years or during pregnancy and lactation. It is not considered appropriate for long term travel, its use generally being limited to up to six months.

Maloprim

Maloprim (a fixed combination of dapsone and pyrimethamine), not to be confused with malarone (see above), is a second-line drug which is sometimes useful where other drugs are unsuitable. The usual adult regimen is chloroquine 300mg with maloprim one tablet, both weekly. The therapeutic ratio is narrow: severe bone marrow toxicity has been reported when two tablets weekly have been taken instead of one. Minor adverse reactions are seen with a similar frequency to other regimens. Caution should be exercised in pregnancy (especially in the first trimester). Maloprim should only be considered during pregnancy where travel to high risk areas is unavoidable and other drugs are unsuitable. Folate supplements are then required.

6.6 Prescribing stand-by therapy

Travellers who will be out of reach of prompt medical attention, particularly in malarious areas where chemoprophylaxis is either not recommended or of limited efficacy, could be provided with a drug regimen to self-treat an episode of malaria. This must be accompanied by careful counselling on the presenting symptoms of malaria, the indications for use of the drug and how to use it safely. If possible, the traveller should try to seek a medical opinion before starting the treatment, but if assistance is not available within eight hours of the onset of symptoms, a full course of therapy should be taken while continuing with other preventive measures. Self-diagnostic tests for falciparum malaria are in development and may be useful in the future for confirming the diagnosis of malaria.

Standby treatment regimen	Usual amount per tablet	Dose
Quinine plus Fansidar	300mg quinine and Fansidar (25mg pyrimethamine + 500mg sulfadoxine)	Quinine 2 tablets 3 times a day for 3 days followed by 3 tablets of Fansidar taken together
Quinine plus doxycycline (or other tetracycline)	300mg quinine, 100mg doxycycline	Quinine 2 tablets 3 times a day for 3 days accompanied by 1 tablet of doxycycline twice daily for 7 days
Malarone	250mg atovaquone + 100mg proguanil	4 tablets once a day for 3 days

Quinine frequently causes adverse reactions such as tinnitus, and people should be forewarned (see page 88 for adverse reations to other drugs).

6.7 Malaria symptoms

Malaria can present any time from about a week to up to a year or more after exposure. Early and rapid diagnosis is necessary to reduce complications and death. All travellers to malarious areas should be advised about the varied symptoms of malaria (see below), which can be non-specific. Travellers should be encouraged to seek medical advice for any new symptoms. Extra doses of chemoprophylactic drugs should be specifically discouraged as this may interfere with diagnosis (and cause adverse reactions). The urgency to make the diagnosis cannot be over-emphasised. Deaths have occurred within 24 hours of the first symptoms. Travellers should be warned that no prophylaxis is 100 per cent effective.

Symptoms of malaria

The symptoms of malaria are usually non-specific. More common symptoms include:
- *Fever, which is the most common symptom*
- *Flu-like illness*
- *Backache*
- *Diarrhoea*
- *Joint pains*
- *Sore throat*
- *Headache*

TABLE 1 Doses of prophylactic antimalarial drugs for adults *

Generic name(s)	Trade names	Usual amount per tablet	Dose for chemoprophylaxis
Chloroquine	Nivaquine, Avloclor	150mg (base)	2 tablets weekly
Proguanil	Paludrine	100mg	2 tablets daily
Mefloquine	Lariam	250mg (228mg in the USA)	1 tablet weekly
Dapsone + Pyrimethamine	Maloprim	100mg + 12.5mg	1 tablet weekly
Atovaquone+ Proguanil	Malarone	250mg+ 100 mg	1 tablet daily
Doxycycline	Vibramycin	100 mg	1 capsule daily

* See BNF for contraindications

TABLE 2 Doses of prophylactic antimalarial drugs for children[†] (in fraction of adult doses)

Weight in kg [††]	Under 6kg	6–9.9kg	10–15.9kg	16–24.9kg	25–44.9kg	45kg and over
Age [††]	Term to 12 weeks	3–11 months	1yr–3yrs 11 months	4yrs–7yrs 11 months	8yrs–12yrs 11 months	13yrs and over
Chloroquine	0.125 dose	0.25 dose	0.375 dose	0.5 dose	0.75 dose	Adult dose
Proguanil	0.125 dose	0.25 dose	0.375 dose	0.5 dose	0.75 dose	Adult dose
Mefloquine	*	0.25 dose	0.25 dose	0.5 dose	0.75 dose	Adult dose
Doxycycline	*	*	*	*	Adult dose	Adult dose
Maloprim [one size]	*	0.25 dose	0.25 dose	0.5 dose	0.75 dose	Adult dose

Caution – in other countries tablet size may vary

* Not recommended

† See BNF for contraindications

†† Weight is a better guide, ages are given as guidelines

TABLE 3 Doses of prophylactic antimalarial drugs for children[†] (in tablets)

Weight in kg[††]	Under 6kg	6–9.9kg	10–15.9kg	16–24.9kg	25–44.9kg	45kg and over
Age[††]	Term to 12 weeks	3–11 months	1yr–3yrs 11 months	4yrs–7yrs 11 months	8yrs–12yrs 11 months	13yrs and over
Chloroquine 150mg base per tablet	$1/4$ tablet	$1/2$ tablet	$3/4$ tablet	1 tablet	$1^1/2$ tablets	2 tablets
Proguanil 100mg per tablet	$1/4$ tablet	$1/2$ tablet	$3/4$ tablet	1 tablet	$1^1/2$ tablets	2 tablets
Mefloquine 250mg	*	$1/4$ tablet	$1/4$ tablet	$1/2$ tablet	$3/4$ tablet	1 tablet
Doxycycline 100mg per capsule	*	*	*	*	1 capsule from 12 yrs	1 capsule
Maloprim [one size]	*	$1/4$ tablet	$1/4$ tablet	$1/2$ tablet	$3/4$ tablet	1 tablet

Caution – in other countries tablet size may vary
* Not recommended
[†] See BNF for contraindications
[††] Weight is a better guide, ages are given as guidelines

TABLE 4 Chloroquine – doses by 5ml spoon measure for children

Weight[††]	Under 4.5 kg	4.5–7.9 kg	8–10.9 kg	11–14.9 kg	15–16.5 kg
Age[††]	Under 6 weeks	6 weeks– 5 months	6 months– 12 months	13 months 2 years 11 months	3 years– 3 years 11 months
Number of 5 ml measures	0.5 (2.5ml)	1 (5ml)	1.5 (5ml + 2.5ml)	2 (5ml + 5ml)	2.5 (5ml + 5ml + 2.5ml)

[††] Weight is a better guide, ages are given as guidelines

7 Arthropod-borne diseases (other than malaria)

A wide range of diseases are transmitted by various arthropod vectors. Many are of great significance to populations residing in the tropics or other endemic zones but are of little risk to the average traveller, although isolated cases may occur. However, cases of dengue fever imported into the UK are increasing. This Chapter includes a table of various arthropod-borne diseases, some information about dengue and the three immunisable diseases (Japanese encephalitis, tick-borne encephailitis and yellow fever) and information on physical methods of protection.

Disease	Type of organism	Vector	Main transmission areas	Vaccination available in the UK?
Bartonellosis/ Oroya fever	Bacterium *Bartonella bacilliformus*	Sandfly	Peru, Ecuador, and Colombia	No
Dengue	Flavivirus	Mosquito	Most tropics and subtropics especially Central and South America (including the Caribbean and Hawaii) SE Asia, S Pacific, and NE Australia	No
Filariasis	Filariae	Mosquito	Sub-Saharan Africa, Egypt, Asia, W Pacific islands, Central America, NE coast of S America and Caribbean	No
Japanese encephalitis	Flavivirus	Mosquito	Across Asia from India to Korea, Japan and SE Asia (and Pakistan); Torres Str Is and some Pacific Is	Yes (unlicensed)
Leishmaniasis	Parasite (Protozoa) *Leishmania*	Sandfly	Tropics and subtropics (including Mediterranean areas)	No
Lyme	Bacterium (spirochete) *Borrelia burgdoferi*	Tick	Temperate areas of Europe and Asia, N/Central and Pacific coast of N America	No (yes in USA for the USA strain)
Onchocerciasis (River blindness)	Filariae	Black fly	Across C Africa, small foci in Yemen, Americas (S Mexico, Brazil, Colombia, Ecuador, Guatemala, Venezuela)	No

Disease	Type of organism	Vector	Main transmission areas	Vaccination available in the UK?
Plague	Bacterium *Yersinia pestis*	Rodent flea	Foci in S America, Western USA, N Africa, East and Southern Africa,Central Asia, India, SE Asia	No
Relapsing fever	Bacterium (spirochete) *Borrelia recurrentis* *7 Borrelia Sp.*	Body and head louse

Tick | Asia, N Africa, Ethiopia and the Sudan, highland areas of C. Africa and S. America
Africa including North and South Middle East, Central Asia, India, and Spain. Also in S. America; sporadic in W. Canada and W. USA. | No |
Rift Valley fever	Phlebovirus	Mosquito	Africa including Egypt, Somalia, Mauritania, Kenya	No
Rocky Mountain spotted fever	Rickettsia	Tick	USA, Canada, Mexico Panama, Costa Rica and Colombia	No
Ross River fever	Toga virus	Mosquito	Australia (South, Victoria, Western, Coast of New South Wales and Queensland) and South Pacific	No
Sandfly fever	Virus Sandfly fever group of viruses	Sandfly	Subtropical and tropical areas of Europe, Middle East, Asia and Africa	No
St Louis encephalitis	Flavivirus	Mosquito	Americas	No
Tick-borne encephalitis	Flavivirus	Tick	C. and eastern Europe and across former USSR to Pacific	Yes
Trypano-somiasis (African sleeping sickness)	Protozoa (Trypanosome) 2 main forms in different parts of Africa *T. gambiense* *T. rhodesiense*	Tsetse fly	East, central and west Africa

Central and west Africa Eastern Africa from Ethiopia, south to Botswana | No |
| Chagas' (American Trypano-somiasis) | Protozoa (Trypanosome) | Reduviid (cone nosed bug) | Americas from Mexico to Argentina | No |

Disease	Type of organism	Vector	Main transmission areas	Vaccination available in the UK?
Tularaemia	Bacterium *Francisella tularensis*	Mosquito Tick, Deerfly*	Parts of continental Europe, Russia, China, Japan, USA.	No
Typhus: **Endemic**	*Rickettsiae* (several spp)	Rat flea	Temperate areas summer months	No
Epidemic		Body louse	Colder months, war/natural disaster, highland areas	
Tick (see also Rocky Mountain spotted fever)		Tick	Africa and Indian subcontinent. Also Mediterranean and E. Europe, Serbia and Australia	
Scrub		Rodent mite	Asia, South Pacific and Australia	
West Nile fever	Flavivirus	Mosquito	Africa, Indian subcontinent, Middle East, former USSR, Europe, one outbreak in 1999 in New York	No
Yellow fever	Flavivirus	Mosquito	West, Central and East Africa, Panama and Tropical south America (see maps inside back cover)	Yes

7.1 Dengue fever/Dengue haemorrhagic fever

Dengue fever (DF) and dengue haemorrhagic fever (DHF) exist throughout most of the tropics and subtropics. There has been a dramatic increase in transmission and cases in recent years with epidemics in tropical South America, the Caribbean and SE Asia and increased cases imported into the UK, from the Caribbean and Thai islands especially.

The four dengue viruses (flaviviruses) are transmitted to man by aedes mosquitoes. The disease may be subclinical or non-specific or have a sudden onset of fever (one to five days), severe headache, joint and muscle aches ('breakbone fever'). A transient early generalised rash may be replaced later by petechiae. Nausea and vomiting may occur.

DF in travellers is usually self-limiting although a return to complete health can sometimes be slow. Immunity is to the type encountered but it is believed that infection with a second type (usually within two years of the first) may result in the more severe DHF which carries a high mortality (particularly in local children) and has occurred in travellers.

There is no specific therapy. Prevention is by reduction of mosquito bites during the day, especially just after dawn and just before dusk (see 7.5).

No vaccine is currently available but several candidate vaccines are under development.

7.2 Japanese encephalitis

Japanese encephalitis (JE) exists only in Asia, from India (and a small area in Pakistan) eastwards across Thailand and China to Korea and Japan and down through south east Asia. It has recently reached the Torres Straight islands between Papua New Guinea and northern Australia.

The flavivirus is transmitted by various species of culicene mosquito from agricultural animals (often pigs) and birds to man. The mosquitoes most commonly breed in rice fields.

The risk season corresponds with the hotter, wetter seasons in the northern part of the endemic zone (usually May–October) whilst it tends to be year round in Malaysia, Indonesia and the Philippines.

The infection is asymptomatic in over 99 per cent of cases. However, when encephalitis develops there is a 30 per cent mortality rate and about 50 per cent of the survivors are left with neurological sequelae.

The disease is extremely rare in travellers, the risk estimated to be less than 0.1 per 100,000 in tourists and business people. It is increased for those staying in rural, especially agricultural, areas within the endemic zone and in the transmission season. Vaccine should be considered for those who will be at this increased risk for at least a month. Prevention for all travellers to rural areas is by reducing the chance of being bitten by these predominantly dusk to dawn biting mosquitoes (see 7.5).

Vaccine (see also *Immunisation against Infectious Disease* and table in Chapter 8)
The unlicensed, inactivated, mouse brain derived vaccine can be administered on a named doctor/named patient basis to those considered at sufficient risk. Possible adverse events include delayed allergic reactions and so the course should be completed at least ten (and preferably 14) days before travel. Vaccinees should be observed for 30 minutes after each dose. Those with a history of urticaria or multiple allergies are considered at higher risk of allergic reactions. Rare neurological reactions also occur.

7.3   Yellow fever

Yellow fever exists within two endemic zones – a belt across Africa and the tropical part of South America reaching as far north as Panama (see maps inside back cover). The risks within these zones will vary according to mosquito activity.

The flavivirus is transmitted by species of aedes and haemagogus mosquitoes in a jungle cycle which includes non-human primates (and occasional humans in the forest) and an urban cycle involving humans.

The disease can be mild, flu-like or hepatitis-like or a severe viral haemorrhagic fever with a 50 to 60 per cent mortality in non-immune travellers.

Prevention is by reducing the chance of mosquito bites from these day biting mosquitoes, especially after dawn and late afternoon (see 7.5) and by vaccine.

Immunisation is advised for all travellers to endemic zones unless travel is restricted to urban areas at high altitude (whether or not it is a mandatory requirement for entry).

Immunisation is available only from designated centres (see pages 3–4).

Vaccine (see also *Immunisation against Infectious Disease* and table in Chapter 8) The live attenuated 17D strain vaccine is highly effective with a very low rate of serious adverse events.

An International Certificate of Vaccination against yellow fever is required for entry to some countries (see 8.2.3).

7.4   Tick-borne encephalitis

Tick-borne encephalitis (TBE) exists in Scandinavia, across Central and Eastern Europe and the Western part of the former USSR. The flavivirus is transmitted by the vector tick *Ixodes ricinus*. A different tick *Ixodes persulcatus* transmits the closely related Russian spring summer encephalitis across the former USSR, north of Mongolia to the Pacific coast and to parts of China (far north east), Korea and Japan. The countries with areas most affected by TBE are Austria, Belarus, Croatia, Czech Republic, Estonia, Germany, Hungary, Latvia, Lithuania, Poland, Russia, Slovakia and Ukraine.

Areas with lower prevalence or where sporadic cases have been reported include Albania, Bulgaria, Denmark (Bornholm Island), SW coast of Finland, France, Greece, Italy, Norway, Romania, Serbia, the Baltic coast of Southern Sweden and Switzerland.

The infection is asymptomatic in 90 per cent of cases especially in children. Those who develop flu-like symptoms may recover but ten per cent of them suffer a relapse with encephalitis with possible neurological sequelae or fatal outcome. The outlook is worse with increasing age.

The risk is mainly to those who are working, walking or camping in rural areas where ticks are prevalent. It is greatest from April through to August and sometimes October. It can extend outside those seasons in the warmer south of the area. The disease is occasionally transmitted by eating or drinking unpasteurised dairy products.

Prevention is by reduction of tick bites, avoidance of consumption of unpasteurised dairy products and by vaccine. The general measures to prevent ticks getting on to skin are described below. Those in tick areas should check their skin for attached ticks, which is easier to do with a partner. Ticks should be removed as soon as possible with tweezers (or fingers covered by tissue paper if no tweezers are available) as close to the skin attachment as possible, by steady pulling without jerking or twisting. Only one to two per cent of ticks are likely to be infected although occasionally up to ten per cent are. Medical advice should be sought locally as specific immunoglobulin may be available and advised within 48 hours (manufacturers state 96 hours) of a tick bite. However its efficacy has been questioned. Immunoglobulin is unlicensed in the UK but can be obtained on a named doctor/named patient basis where it is believed to be beneficial.

Vaccine (see also *Immunisation against Infectious Disease* and table in Chapter 8) Inactivated vaccines are available in the UK for those considered at risk. Ideally immunisation should be completed at least a month before travel. It is considered to be effective against both strains of the disease. The specific immunoglobulin may on occasion be considered for those at high risk and travelling at short notice, although it is unlicensed in the UK.

Experience with TBE vaccine in the UK is limited. Adverse reactions including tenderness and swelling at the injection site with regional lymph gland swelling are reported, with some more generalised malaise, limb aches and pyrexia in some cases. Neuritis is rarely reported.

7.5 Physical methods of protection against mosquito and tick-borne diseases

For the prevention of bites from night time (dusk-dawn) biting mosquitoes see paragraph 6.4. For day time biting mosquitoes this advice applies dawn to dusk. In practice this will often include sleeping time.

Tick bites are reduced by preventing vegetation from brushing against bare skin, which should therefore be covered eg long trousers tucked into socks. Open sandals should not be worn. DEET based repellents have some action against ticks and can be used on skin or to spray clothing. Permethrin insecticide spray can also be used on clothes. (See previous page for removal of ticks).

Immunisation for overseas travel

8.1   Introduction

Immunisation requirements for international travel are often the primary health concern of both prospective travellers and their doctors, usually followed by the choice of malaria tablet.

Immunisation is only one part of health advice for travellers. Attendance for immunisation provides an opportunity to deliver further health protection information on, for example, prevention of accidents and travellers' diarrhoea (Chapters 4 and 5), or specific advice relevant to the individual traveller.

The disease risk for the individual traveller should be assesed, as far as is possible, when choosing travel vaccines. The risk to a business traveller, for example, visiting only the most hygienic, air-conditioned premises for a few days should not be equated with that for someone travelling extensively to rural areas of the same country where not only is the risk to health increased but the facilities for medical treatment are likely to be less developed. The information on which to base such decisions is sometimes inadequate, not least because of limited reporting from some of the geographical areas of greatest risk. Some risks may be seasonal, or limited to certain geographical areas, and many are influenced by personal lifestyle or occupation, eg the risk for hepatitis B and HIV (Chapter 9). The risk of vaccine preventable disease for package holiday travel will depend on the itinerary and on the behaviour of the individuals involved, but will often be low.

Travellers may be informed by travel companies or embassies that "no vaccinations/immunisations are needed" or "nothing is needed" for a certain destination, and may omit to seek further medical advice. Education of travellers should include the information that "nothing needed" may mean no certificates are officially required but that **optional** immunisations, usually more important for personal health protection, may be advised in addition to other health-related precautions.

8.2   International Certificates of Vaccination

The International Health Regulations adopted by the World Health Organization were devised to help prevent the international spread of diseases and, in the context of international travel, to do so with the minimum of inconvenience to the passenger (WHO, International Travel and Health 2000).

It should be remembered that the Regulations are more a public health measure for the receiving country than for protection of the individual.

8.2.1 Yellow Fever

Yellow fever is now the only disease for which an international vaccination certificate may be required for entry into a country. Many countries (not the UK) require a valid International Certificate of Vaccination from travellers arriving from, or who have been in transit through, yellow fever infected areas or countries with infected areas. The maps inside the back page show the "yellow fever endemic zones" where there is a potential risk of infection. Some countries consider these zones as "infected" areas for the purpose of International Certificate of Vaccination requirements. Other countries require a certificate from all entering travellers. Details of requirements are included in the entries for individual countries (Chapter 3). They are published annually in International Travel and Health, Vaccination Requirements and Health Advice (WHO). Failure to provide a valid certificate to the port health authorities could, in some circumstances, result in a traveller being immunised, denied entry or quarantined.

The International Certificate is valid for ten years beginning ten days after the vaccination date; this should be entered with the month written in letters. It should be signed by the person authorised by the national health administration (a stamp alone is not acceptable) and by the patient (or parent/guardian). (NB. All the partners in a practice which is a Yellow Fever Vaccination Centre are deemed by the Department of Health to be authorised persons). The manufacturer and batch number of the vaccine and the official stamp of the centre must also be included in the correct space provided.

If a physician advises that an individual should not be immunised on medical grounds, including infants under nine months of age, an exemption certificate may be provided (Appendix 1).

Yellow fever vaccination is recommended for travel to all countries in the endemic zones, whether or not an international certificate is required, and especially if rural areas will be visited. (See country by country advice).

8.2.2 Yellow Fever Designated Centres

Yellow fever vaccine may be administered only at centres which are designated by the national health administration and recorded with WHO. This is to ensure that vaccine storage, administration and certification is carried out correctly. (The current UK list of designated centres is available from http://tap.ccta.gov.uk/doh/yellcode. nsf/pages/Home?open, together with information for practices wishing to apply for designation.)

8.2.3   Cholera

In 1973, the International Health Regulations were amended so that **no country should require a certificate of vaccination against cholera** (WHO, International Travel & Health 1994). This followed acceptance that cholera vaccination does not prevent introduction of the infection into a country. Many countries continued to require proof of cholera immunisation long after 1973, but gradually the present position has been reached where there are no official requirements.

Until recently unofficial demands at a few international air and sea ports resulted in travellers continuing to request immunisation for certification. Reports of such incidents are now extremely rare, and appear to be confined to remote land borders in areas where there have been recent cholera outbreaks.

The conventional parenteral vaccine provided poor protection and is no longer available in the UK. In the rare circumstance where an unofficial demand may be anticipated, confirmation of non-requirement of cholera vaccine may be given on official notepaper signed and stamped by the medical practitioner (Appendix 1). Some new generation cholera vaccines are marketed in certain European countries.

Most travellers are at extremely low risk of contracting cholera. Prevention is by food and water hygiene (see Chapter 5).

8.2.4   Meningococcal vaccination for the pilgrimage to Mecca

Saudi Arabia requires pilgrims to produce proof of immunisation against meningococcal infection issued not more than three years and not less than ten days before arrival in the country. Details are listed in the Saudi Arabia entry (see also important information at 8.4.4).

8.3 Vaccines

Live vaccines	Inactivated vaccines
Measles ⎫ Mumps ⎬ and MMR Rubella ⎭ Oral poliomyelitis Oral typhoid BCG (TB) Yellow fever	Diphtheria toxoid ⎫ Tetanus toxoid ⎬ and combination vaccines Pertussis ⎭ Poliomyelitis (injectable) Haemophilus influenza b (Hib) Influenza Pneumococcal Hepatitis A ⎫ and combination vaccines Hepatitis B ⎭ Typhoid Injectable (and hepatitis A combined vaccine) Meningococcal (A&C) Japanese encephalitis Tick-borne encephalitis Rabies

Doses and recommended schedules are summarised on pages 97 to 108. Information about individual vaccines is contained in the current edition of the memorandum Immunisation against Infectious Disease.

8.4 Recommendations

These are contained in the invidual country entries in Chapter 3. They assume that childhood immunisations, including BCG, are up to date.

8.4.1 Routine immunisations

All individuals should have completed primary tetanus, diphtheria and poliomyelitis courses. A full course comprises five doses of each. When over ten years has elapsed since the primary course and travel is to a developing area a tetanus booster should be given; a diptheria booster should also be given if travel is for more than one month. The appropriate combined diptheria/tetanus preparation is now normally used when either of these is due. A polio booster may be advised for travel to certain countries if ten years has elapsed since the primary course (see country by country advice).

8.4.2 Influenza and pneumococcal vaccines

Those who are recommended to have influenza or pneumococcal vaccine as part of UK policy are advised to be immunised before travel.

8.4.3 Hepatitis A

Where hepatitis A protection is recommended for travel, vaccine is the preferred option rather than normal immunoglobulin. There is some evidence of protection even when vaccine is given after exposure, so that if time before departure is short, the vaccine is still considered likely to prevent or at least modify the infection.

8.4.4 Meningococcal vaccine

Conjugate meningococcal C vaccine (MenC) has recently been introduced into the routine UK childhood immunisation programme. This vaccine protects only against group C meningococcal infection, while much meningococcal infection abroad is caused by Group A. The currently used vaccine for travel is therefore meningococcal A&C polysaccharide vaccine.

A quadravalent vaccine, also containing Y and W135 strains, is now more widely available and is the recommended vaccine for all pilgrims to Saudi Arabia.

Some mild urticarial reactions have been reported in children given A&C vaccine shortly after MenC vaccine. It is not known whether this rate is higher than could be expected with A&C alone, but an interval of two weeks is recommended if A&C vaccine is required following MenC. Until further evidence emerges it is also currently recommended that where MenC vaccine is due following A&C vaccine, the MenC vaccine is delayed until six months after A&C vaccine. In high risk situations, however, MenC vaccine should not be delayed. The local Consultant in Communicable Disease Control or Immunisation Co-ordinator should be consulted.

8.4.5 Combination vaccines

Combination travel vaccines are now available containing more than one vaccine in one preparation, such as adult diphtheria and tetanus. Vaccines recommended should be appropriate for the individual. Where a recipient requires protection against both diseases, at least for the early doses, a combination preparation can be useful.

However, where the two components of a combination (eg hepatitis A with hepatitis B or hepatitis A with typhoid) are not both indicated for the individual traveller, the combined vaccine should not replace the individual vaccines. Where the individual components differ in duration of immunity or number of doses required to complete the course, combined vaccines can also complicate scheduling. Single antigen vaccines may be required for boosters.

Modern vaccines and sharp needles produce little discomfort when skilfully administered and many recipients are unable to report the exact number of injections received.

8.4.6 Infants and small children travelling

Routine infant immunisations may be advised earlier than normally scheduled when children are travelling to high-risk countries for prolonged periods and may have close contact with the indigenous population (for example staying with relatives abroad). In particular, earlier immunisation may be advised if travel is so prolonged that routine childhood immunisations would be delayed.

Hepatitis B vaccine and BCG can be given from birth where indicated. Polio can, if necessary, be commenced from birth, but an extra dose is then advised later on; DTP-Hib can be administered from six weeks of age. Children over six months of age who have not yet received their first dose of MMR, travelling to visit relatives in a measles endemic area, should be offered MMR. However two further doses of MMR are then recommended: one as soon as practicable after the first birthday and the normal pre school booster.

Hepatitis A is usually a mild disease in young children, and infection results in lifelong immunity. Vaccine is therefore often considered unnecessary in this age group (although opinions differ). It is more likely to be considered for those travelling to visit friends and relatives for longer periods in areas of high endemicity. There is an argument that the children should be immunised to prevent secondary infection in non-immune adult contacts of the children, eg play group leaders, on their return.

The addition of conjugate meningococcal group C vaccine (MenC) to the routine schedule may result in a small child travelling to, for example, Africa requiring the A&C vaccine close to the new vaccine (see 8.4.4).

The table of immunisations (pages 94–104) provides the lower age limit for travel vaccines where these are specified and the varying ages at which the paediatric dose changes to the adult dose.

8.5   Schedules

Wherever possible, the recommended intervals between doses and between vaccines should be followed and time allowed for antibody to be produced, courses completed and any reaction to have dissipated before the date of travel.

In theory each travel vaccine should be given at least ten days (and preferably three weeks) from another in order to identify the source of any reaction. In practice, time constraints, travel dates and sheer practicality have resulted in many vaccines being given simultaneously without apparent adverse effects.

8.5.1   Live Vaccines

Live vaccines should be administered at least three weeks apart or on the same day. However, the two oral vaccines, typhoid and polio, are usually separated (by at least two weeks) on the theoretical grounds of possible interference in the gut. There is no evidence to preclude oral typhoid being given with yellow fever or human normal immunoglobulin (HNIG).

Live virus vaccines may suppress the tuberculin test and so should be delayed until after the test has been read.

8.5.2   Inactivated Vaccines

Inactivated vaccines can be given simultaneously with any other vaccine, but at a different site, the number given taking into account the comfort of the patient. Concurrent administration of vaccines can make it difficult to elucidate adverse reactions. An exception to the simultaneous administration rule concerns meningococcal A&C and the recently introduced conjugate meningococcal C vaccine (see Meningococcal vaccine 8.4.4).

8.5.3   Human Normal Immunoglobulin (see 8.4.3)

The antibody response to MMR (or measles, mumps or rubella given separately) could be inhibited by HNIG which should be delayed until three weeks after the vaccine. If HNIG has already been given, three months should elapse before giving MMR.

HNIG has **not** been shown to inhibit yellow fever, oral typhoid or BCG and any effect it has on OPV is unlikely to be significant where the OPV is a booster.

HNIG is anyway usually given after the vaccines and closer to the departure date because of its rapid efficacy and shorter duration of action.

8.5.4   Timing

Courses of most travel vaccines, plus the single dose vaccines, can be administered over a four week period. The final doses should ideally be completed a little ahead of the departure date to allow immunity to develop. It can take up to four weeks, for instance, for full immunity to develop following Japanese encephalitis vaccine. (This vaccine is anyway recommended to be completed at least ten, and preferably 14, days prior to travel because of the possibility of a delayed allergic reaction.)

More time will be required if a primary course of tetanus, polio or diphtheria is necessary. If the full course cannot be completed before departure, it is usually worth giving the maximum number of doses that the travel departure date allows, completing the course on return.

Travellers should be encouraged to plan to start immunisations well in advance of travel.

Vaccines for Overseas Travel (See *Immunisation against Infectious Disease* for further detail and page 161 for vaccine manufacturers)

Vaccine and age given	Primary course	Interval between doses	Reinforcing doses	Comments
BCG				
Celltech Medeva From birth	Single dose, 0.1ml id (0.05ml <3/12 of age) after Heaf testing (except for neonates)	N/A	None	Given only if no BCG scar and skin test negative
Diphtheria				
Adsorbed diphtheria vaccine, child – Celltech Medeva				
<10 years	3 doses (usually as DTP), 0.5ml sc or im	4 weeks	At school entry or 3 years after last dose	
Adult low dose diphtheria vaccine – Distributed by Farillon (as part of the National Childhood Immunisation Programme)				
>10 years	3 doses, 0.5ml sc or im	4 weeks	At school leaving (as Td) or 10 years after primary course	see 8.4.1
Diphtheria and Tetanus vaccine for adults and adolescents (Td)				
Diftavax Aventis Pasteur MSD > 10 years	3 doses, 0.5 ml deep sc or im	4 weeks	After 10 years	see 8.4.1

8

Hepatitis A – vaccine

Vaccine and age given	Primary course	Interval between doses	Reinforcing doses	Comments
Avaxim **Aventis Pasteur MSD** 16 years and over	Single dose, 0.5ml im		Booster at 6–12 months predicted to provide antibodies which persist for at least 10 years	
Havrix Monodose **Glaxo Smith Kline** 16 years and over	Single dose, 1ml im		Booster after 6–12 months to provide long-term antibody titres (5–10 years)	
Havrix Junior Monodose **Glaxo Smith Kline** 1–15 years	Single dose, 0.5ml im		Booster after 6-12 months provides immunity for up to 10 years	see 8.4.6
Vaqta Adult **Aventis Pasteur MSD** 18 years and over	Single dose, 1ml im		Booster after 6–12 months: 'long-term duration of serum antibodies to hepatitis A virus unknown'	
Vaqta Paediatric **Aventis Pasteur MSD** 2 years up to and including 17years	Single dose, 0.5ml im		Booster at 6–18 months: 'long term duration of serum antibody to hepatitis A virus unknown'	see 8.4.6

Vaccine and age given	Primary course	Interval between doses	Reinforcing doses	Comments
Hepatitis A – Immunoglobulin (see 8.3)				
Gammabulin **Baxter Hyland Immuno** **Kabiglobulin** (when available) **Pharmacia and Upjohn**				
<10 Years	Single injection 125mg for 2 months protection; 250mg for 3–5 months protection			For single short trips
<10 Years	250mg for 2 months protection; 500mg for 3–5 months protection			For single short trips
Hepatitis A + Hepatitis B combined				
Twinrix Adult **Smith Kline Glaxo** 16 years and older	3 doses, 1ml im	0, 1 and 6 months	Booster with combined vaccine recommended 5 years after initiation of primary course. If monovalent vaccines used as booster: hepatitis A – administer after 10 years; hepatitis B administer after 5 years	

Vaccine and age given	Primary course	Interval between doses	Reinforcing doses	Comments
Twinrix Paediatric **Glaxo Smith Kline** 1 year up to and including 15 years	3 doses, 0.5ml im	0,1 and 6 months	As for Twinrix Adult	
Hepatitis A + Typhoid combined				
Hepatyrix **Glaxo Smith Kline** 15 years and over	Single dose, 1ml im		Booster of hepatitis A at 6-12 months. Single dose of Vi polysaccharide vaccine every 3 years.	
Hepatitis B				
Engerix B **Glaxo Smith Kline**	3 doses, adults and chidren over 15 years, 1ml (20mg) im; neonates and children 15 years and under, 0.5ml (10mg) im	0, 1 and 6 months	'Not known whether responders will need booster doses'	For more rapid immunisation the third dose may be given at 2 months and a booster at 12 months. Accelerated schedule for Engerix B in those 18 years and over: 0, 7 and 21 days with a reinforcing dose at 12 months

Vaccine and age given	Primary course	Interval between doses	Reinforcing doses	Comments
HB Vax II **Aventis Pasteur MSD** 16 years and over	3 doses, 1ml im	0, 1 and 6 months or 0, 1, 2 and 12 months	'Need for booster not yet defined'	Accelerated schedule (0, 1, 2 and12 months) may induce protective antibody levels earlier
HB Vax II Paediatric **Aventis Pasteur MSD** Birth through to and including 15 years	3 doses, 0.5ml	0, 1 and 6 months or 0, 1, 2 and 12 months	As for HB Vax II	As for HB Vax II
Influenza				
Various manufacturers Check individual manufacturers' current data sheet	Dose will vary according to age		For risk groups: annual immunisation with vaccine containing the most recent strains	Influenza vaccine is prepared annually from strains recommended for that year by the World Health Organization

Japanese encephalitis

NB: Two dose schedules are included in the data sheet; however in non-immune travellers, 3 doses are usually advised for optimum protection. Complete course at least 10–14 days pre-travel.

Vaccine and age given	Primary course	Interval between doses	Reinforcing doses	Comments
Biken, manufactured in Japan and distributed by Aventis Pasteur MSD				
<3 years (but no data <1 year)	3 doses, 0.5 ml sc or 2 doses, 0.5 ml sc	0, 7 and 30 days 0, 7 days	Booster after 2–4 years Booster after 3 months	Unlicensed vaccine. Where 3 doses impossible, 2dose regimen provides immunity for 3 months in 80% of recipients. Manufacturer states that 0, 7, 14 days schedule may be used where urgent.
>3 years	3 doses, 1.0 ml sc or 2 doses, 1.0 ml sc	0, 7 and 30 days 0, 7 days	Booster after 2–4 years Booster after 3 months	
Green Cross, manufactured in Korea and distributed by MASTA	2 doses	0, 7–14 days	Booster after 1 year and then 3 years (annually if at high risk)	Unlicensed vaccine. See note above

Meningococcal

Vaccine and age given	Primary course	Interval between doses	Reinforcing doses	Comments
ACWY Vax GlaxoSmithKline >2 years	Single dose, 0.5ml deep sc			Children aged 2 months to 2 years may get short lived response to the A, W_{135} and Y antigens
AC Vax GlaxoSmithKline >2 months	Single dose, 0.5ml deep sc or im		In adults and children > 5 years, immunity will persist for up to 5 years. In younger children, particularly those < 2 years, immunity against group C meningitis is unlikely to persist for more than 1 or 2 years	8.4.4
Mengivac A+C Aventis Pasteur MSD >18 months	Single dose, 0.5ml deep sc or im		Post vaccination immunity lasts at least 3 years	8.4.4

Vaccine and age given	Primary course	Interval between doses	Reinforcing doses	Comments
Pneumococcal				
Pneumovax II Aventis Pasteur MSD 2 years and above	Single dose, 0.5ml sc or im		Re-vaccination is not usually recommended, except for individuals in whom antibody levels are likely to have declined more rapidly (see 10.3)	
Poliomyelitis				
OPV Distributed by Farillon as part of the National Childhood Immunisation Programme	3 doses	4 weeks	Children at entry and before leaving school Adults 10 yearly if at continuing risk	Faecal excretion of vaccine virus up to 6 weeks. May be longer if immuno suppressed.
IPV Distributed by Farillon	3 doses, 0.5ml sc or im	4 weeks	As above	Unlicensed vaccine; named patients only

Vaccine and age given	Primary course	Interval between doses	Reinforcing doses	Comments
Rabies Pre-exposure				
Aventis Pasteur MSD (human diploid cell vaccine)				
No lower age stated	3 doses, 1.0ml sc or im or 0.1 ml id	0, 7 and 28 days	2–3 years if at continued exposure	Id route is unlicensed
	2 doses, 1.0ml sc or im or 0.1 ml id	0 and 28 days	Booster at 6–12 months then 2–3 years	Most, but not all, individuals seroconvert after 2 doses. May be acceptable for travellers who are not animal handlers
Rabipur (purified chick embryo cell vaccine) Chiron distributed by MASTA	3 doses, 1.0ml im	0, 7 and 21 or 28 days	Generally every 2–5 years (see manufacturer's information)	

Vaccine and age given	Primary course	Interval between doses	Reinforcing doses	Comments
Tetanus				
Celltech Medeva				
<10 years (usual childhood course)	3 doses usually as DTP, 0.5ml sc or im	4 weeks	At school entry or 3 years after last dose	
>10 years	3 doses adsorbed vaccine or as Td 0.5ml sc or im	4 weeks	At school leaving (as Td) or 10 years after primary course; further booster 10 years later	
Tick-borne encephalitis – vaccine				
Ticovac **Baxter Hyland Immuno** >36 months	3 doses, 0.5ml im (the first dose should be 0.25ml for children 36 months to 15 years) or 2 doses, 0.5 ml im (the first dose should be 0.25ml for children 36 months to 15 years)	0, 21 days–3 months, then 9–12 months 0 and 14 days, then 1 year	Booster after 3 years	Vaccine licensed Spring 2000 Protection after 2 doses lasts 12 months.
FSME-Immuno **Baxter Hyland Immuno** No lower age limit given	3 doses 0.5 ml sc or im or 2 doses, 0.5 ml sc or im	0, 4–12 weeks then, 9–12 months 0 and 14 days	Booster after 3 years	Unlicensed vaccine named patients only 2 dose regimen gives immunity for one year

Vaccine and age given	Primary course	Interval between doses	Reinforcing doses	Comments
Encepur Chiron (distributed by MASTA) 12 years and over	3 doses, 0.5ml im	0, 4 weeks then 9–12 months or, 0, 7, 21 days then 12–18 months	Booster after 3 years	Unlicensed vaccine – for named patients only
Tick-borne encephalitis – immunoglobulin				
FSME-BULIN Baxter Hyland Immuno	Single dose, dependent on body weight			Unlicensed. Rarely considered for pre-exposure, may be considered for post-exposure (see 7.4)
Typhoid				
Typherix GlaxoSmithKline > 2 years	Single dose, 0.5 ml im		Single dose every 3 years	
Typhim Vi Aventis Pasteur MSD > 18 months	Single dose, 0.5ml deep sc or im		Single dose every 3 years	

Vaccine and age given	Primary course	Interval between doses	Reinforcing doses	Comments
Typhoid				
Vivotif Live, oral Strain Ty21a (distributed by MASTA) > 6 years	3 doses of one capsule	Alternate days	Full 3 dose course annually	Remind recipient of appropriate storage (in fridge)

Hepatyrix (combined hepatitis A + typhoid) - see under Hepatitis A vaccine

Yellow fever				
Celltech Medeva > 9 months	Single dose, 0.5 ml sc		10 yearly	Given at designated centres only

Sexually transmitted and blood-borne infections, including HIV and hepatitis B, and overseas travel

9.1   Introduction

Unprotected sexual activity overseas even during short holidays, places an individual at risk of transmission of sexually transmitted infections including human immunodeficiency virus (HIV) and hepatitis B. Sexually transmitted infections are endemic world-wide, but much more prevalent in certain overseas destinations. Prevalence of HIV in the UK is highest in gay/bisexual men. However, in 1999 for the first time, newly reported HIV infections acquired heterosexually exceeded those in gay/bisexual men. Most of these heterosexually acquired infections were acquired whilst living abroad, mainly in sub-Saharan African countries.

AIDS cases have been reported from every country in the world, including those in Europe (in 1998 thirteen countries in Europe had incidence levels of HIV infection higher than the UK). In general, the prevalence of HIV infection is highest in groups with high levels of risk behaviour for infection (eg homosexual men, persons with many sexual partners, sex workers, injecting drug users) who are usually to be found in urban areas. In some cities in the highest risk countries of the world, most of which are in sub-Saharan Africa and South East Asia, as many as one in four young and middle-aged adults in the general population may be infected with the virus.

Hepatitis B infection exists world-wide. Countries of low prevalence include north and Westren Europe, North America, Australia and New Zealand, although prevalence is higher in groups with high risk behaviour. Intermediate prevalence areas include Eastern Europe, North Africa, the Indian subcontinent and parts of Central and South America. High prevalence areas include most of sub-Saharan Africa, the Far East and the Pacific Islands. The risk of infection for short term travellers is generally low, provided they do not put themselves at risk by their behaviour or unless blood transfusion is required.

Hepatitis C is endemic in every continent, with a higher prevalence in some countries in Africa, the Middle East, South East Asia and the Western Pacific. In developed countries, routine screening of blood for transfusion (and blood products and organ tissues) has virtually eliminated this route of transmission, sharing contaminated needles now being the most common route. Many developing countries still use unscreened blood and blood products.

9.2 Prevention

9.2.1 Sexual intercourse

It is imperative that travellers
- are aware that a person infected with an STI, HIV or hepatitis B may appear to be perfectly healthy and may not even know they are infected
- avoid unprotected sexual intercourse with anyone other than a regular partner
- always use good quality condoms – this will reduce the likelihood of acquiring other STIs as well as HIV (condoms purchased abroad may be of poor quality)
- carry condoms rather than try to obtain them at the last minute
- appreciate that sex tourism (travel to a country with the explicit intention of having sex, commercial or otherwise, with men or women in that country) is hazardous. It has particularly been a source of infection with HIV and other STIs among UK residents travelling to Thailand
- remember that alcohol weakens inhibitions and makes precautions more easily forgotten

9.2.2 Intravenous drug abuse and body piercing

Travellers should also be aware of;
- the risk of sharing equipment for administering drugs
- the dangers of any procedure which punctures the skin (eg tattooing, ear-piercing) as the sterility of instruments cannot be guaranteed

Using or carrying illicit drugs abroad can also attract very severe penalties.

9.2.3 Medical care

Injections: Standards of infection control in some countries may be inadequate to prevent the spread of blood-borne infections such as hepatitis B and C and HIV. Instruments may not be sterilised between patients and needles and syringes may be re-used. It may be helpful for travellers to carry a clearly labelled medical kit containing sterile sutures, syringes and needles for use in an emergency. Those on group expeditions should consider including a plasma expander in the kit.

Blood transfusions: Not all countries screen all blood donated for transfusion. Travellers should avoid transfusion unless absolutely required and ensure as far as possible that blood they are given has been screened for HIV antibodies. The nearest British Consulate may be able to give advice.

Insurance: Medical insurance should cover the cost of all contingencies, including evacuation in an emergency.

9.2.4 Hepatitis B vaccine

Hepatitis B vaccine may be indicated in addition to the above precautions, in particular for longer stay travellers and shorter term travellers who may place themselves at risk from their behaviour.

10 Respiratory diseases and travel

10.1 Introduction

Respiratory infections are common both at home and abroad and frequently affect people while travelling. Certain situations which may be encountered when travelling, and certain infections, place the traveller at some increased risk of a respiratory infection.

10.2 Acute respiratory infections

Some travellers spend considerable periods in crowded conditions or communal living which may increase the risk of acute respiratory infections such as colds, influenza and bronchitis. Most are self-limiting virus infections for which there is no specific treatment. If symptoms persist or worsen, medical attention should be sought. Practitioners should be aware that respiratory pathogens acquired abroad may have unusual antimicrobial resistance patterns.

10.3 Influenza and pneumococcal infections

Influenza infection occurs throughout the world mainly in winter (it should be remembered that in the southern hemisphere this is during the summer months of the northern hemisphere). In the tropics, influenza activity is not seasonal. For most travellers no specific protection against influenza is recommended and treatment should be symptomatic. Influenza immunisation before travel should be considered for individuals for whom annual influenza immunisation is recommended in the UK, such as those (of any age) with certain chronic underlying diseases and those aged 65 and over.

The risk of pneumococcal infection is increased in certain groups and increases with age; high altitude may add to the risk. Immunisation is advised for those at increased risk in accordance with the recommendations in *Immunisation against Infectious Disease*.

10.4 Legionnaires' disease

Legionnaires' disease is an uncommon form of pneumonia or severe chest infection which has a significant mortality, particularly among middle aged or elderly adults. It may be contracted anywhere in the world. Both sporadic cases and outbreaks of legionnaires' disease have been reported among holiday makers who have stayed in hotels and apartment blocks, particularly around the Mediterranean. Although the risk for any individual is extremely small, the diagnosis should be considered in travellers who develop a respiratory illness, particularly pneumonia, during or on return from their travel, so that appropriate treatment can be instituted promptly. No preventive measures against acquiring legionnaires' disease are available to the individual.

Use of a rapid diagnostic test (e.g. detection of antigen in urine) will enable rapid and appropriate antibiotic treatment to be given, thus reducing the risk of severe illness and death from this disease.

10.5 Tuberculosis

Tuberculosis (TB) is one of the major global public health challenges. The World Health Organization estimates that one third of the world's population is infected with TB, and it is the major cause of death from a single infectious agent among adults in the developing world. There has been some increase in TB in parts of the industrialised world.

In many countries of Africa and Asia, infection with HIV has further increased morbidity and mortality from TB: TB is responsible for about 40 per cent of AIDS-related deaths in Africa. Drug resistant TB is increasing in many areas of the world.

Among travellers from industrialised countries, the families of migrants returning to visit relatives abroad are particularly at risk. The risk for other travellers is limited as transmission of the infection usually requires prolonged close contact.

Regions of the world can be categorised based on the incidence of cases of tuberculosis reported to the World Health Organization. The incidence of tuberculosis is generally high in Africa, Asia and South America and low in industrialised countries. Some countries within global regions may, however, have incidence rates that differ substantially from that seen in the rest of their region. For countries in low risk regions, with an incidence rate of up to 40 per 100,000 population, no specific recommendation for BCG immunisation is made for travellers. For countries defined as high risk (incidence rate over 40 per 100,000 population), BCG is recommended for visits longer than about a month, particularly if living or working with the local population. (See under disease risks for each area for the risk for particular countries).

BCG should only be offered to those not previously immunised and who have a negative tuberculin skin test (see *Immunisation against Infectious Disease* for further details).

11 Environmental hazards: heat, cold and altitude

11.1 Ultraviolet radiation

Around 40,000 people in the UK develop skin cancer each year, a figure which is rising by five to six per cent annually. Between 1989 and 1998, deaths from malignant melanoma rose by 35 per cent. This upward trend is believed to be due to the increased extent to which people with mainly white skin expose themselves to ultraviolet radiation (UVR), primarily sunlight, but probably also from sun beds and similar devices. Much exposure, is associated with foreign travel and summer holidays.

While the sun should be enjoyed, advice on sunbathing should clearly take account of the risks as well as the benefits and overexposure at times when ultraviolet intensity is high should be avoided.

11.1.1 Those most at risk include:

- babies and children
- those with pale skin which sunburns easily, fair or red hair, freckles or with over 50 normal moles or with a family history of malignant melanoma
- dedicated sun worshippers
- outdoor workers

For people with brown or black skin the risk of sun induced skin cancer is minimal, although skin photoageing still fairly readily occurs.

11.1.2 What to advise

The UK Skin Cancer Prevention Working Party has estimated that at least four out of every five skin cancers are preventable and issued the following statements:

1. There is increasing evidence that excessive sun exposure, and particularly sunburn when aged under 15, is a major risk factor for skin cancer in later life. Protection of the skin of children and adolescents is therefore particularly important.
2. Sun induced skin damage is cumulative.
3. Sun exposure giving rise to sunburn and subsequent skin damage can take place even in the UK.
4. Those who have an outdoor occupation and those with an outdoor recreation such as golf, gardening, skiing or sailing, are also at risk and should learn to protect their skin.

5. A tan is a sign that already damaged skin is trying to protect itself from further damage.
6. To minimise sun induced skin damage:
   - Avoid noonday sun (between 11.00am and 3pm).
   - Seek natural shade in the form of trees or other shelter.
   - Use clothing as a sunscreen including T-shirts, long-sleeved shirts and hats.
   - Use a broad spectrum sun screen with an SPF of 15 or higher to protect against UVB, and with UVA protection.

11.1.3 Sunbeds

Those who use sunbeds either before travel or as a regular exercise should be advised that they emit ultraviolet radiation which is likely to age the skin prematurely and increase the risk of skin cancers. Those under 16 years old, people who burn easily or tan poorly, those taking photosensitising drugs and those with a strong family history of skin cancer should be advised not to use them at all.

11.2 Heatstroke

A separate risk of overexposure to the sun, particularly overseas, is sunstroke or heatstroke, caused simply by overheating. People acclimatise to the heat. Taking it easy for the first few days of exposure is important and strenuous exercise should be avoided. Once acclimatised, water requirements increase rather than decrease and an adequate fluid intake (of non-alcoholic 'safe' liquids) is still of major importance to balance the loss of body fluid through perspiration. For those eating a normal diet, extra salt is **not** advised.

11.3 Cold

11.3.1 The major risks to people exposed to the cold are:

- local cooling, primarily affecting the hands and feet which may freeze (frostbite) or remain cold but unfrozen for long periods (non-freezing cold injury or "trenchfoot" which primarily affects the feet);
- general body cooling leading to hypothermia.

Those at greatest risk are the ill prepared.

Frostbite can occur in anyone exposed to temperatures below freezing without adequate protection to the extremities, and **non-freezing cold injury** can occur where the feet are cold (and generally wet) for extended periods. Visitors to cold climates should be aware of the symptoms of **hypothermia**, which can include subtle mood changes, stumbling and apparent tiredness.

Prevention is by the provision of appropriate clothing including hat, gloves/mittens, suitable socks and boots. Loss of articles of clothing in an accident can be disastrous unless spares are carried. There is an abundance of excellent protective clothing available; fashion should not override safety. If there is the slightest risk that the individual may need to camp out, food rations and a sleeping bag should be carried.

Specialist advice should be sought as to the best equipment for a trip, including a survival bag.

Treatment of someone suffering from hypothermia entails preventing any further drop in body temperature. This should involve seeking shelter and insulating and protecting the victim. Metallised plastic sheeting (space blanket) is ineffective in field conditions and conventional plastic bags (which eliminate evaporative heat loss) are more effective and practical. Great care should be taken in evacuation and rapid rewarming should be avoided unless the individual is well and conscious. Frostbite should not be defrosted if there is a likelihood of re-freezing occurring as this will greatly exacerbate the problem.

11.4 Altitude

Cold is a factor generally experienced at altitude, and the risks and precautions that need to be taken follow those given above.

Altitude-induced illnesses include Acute Benign Mountain Sickness, the symptoms of which include headache, nausea, dizziness, loss of appetite, vomiting and insomnia, which can progress to Acute High Altitude Pulmonary and Cerebral Oedema, a life threatening disorder which most frequently occurs following a rapid ascent to high altitude.

Avoidance of these conditions is best achieved by maximising the opportunity to acclimatise and this should be built into the itinerary. The appearance of any symptoms of Acute Mountain Illness should prompt consideration of descent, or at least the decision to go no higher until they resolve. Continued symptoms should trigger a timely shift to a lower altitude.

Prophylaxis: for susceptible travellers, or when time for natural acclimatisation is limited, prophylactic acetazolamide has been effective in preventing altitude illness, but it has not been shown to protect against cerebral or pulmonary oedema. Paraesthesiae in the fingers and toes are common during the first two days of treatment; sulphonamide allergy, and impaired renal function are contraindications to its use.

Dangerous bites and stings

12.1   Bites by dogs and other large mammals

Bites by dogs are common in all parts of the world. They may cause mechanical damage, including soft tissue injury, avulsion of nerves and tendons, compound fractures, and, rarely, death. They may also be complicated by a range of bacterial infections including tetanus. Some infections are peculiar to animal bites (eg Pasteurella multocida and rabies).

Bites may also be inflicted by domestic cats and monkeys, and less commonly by horses, rodents, bats and even large carnivores.

Infection may occasionally be introduced through scratches and licks over broken skin.

12.1.1 Treatment

Animal bites should not be ignored. Travellers should be advised to:
- clean the wound thoroughly as soon as possible with soap/detergent and water (preferably under a running tap)
- apply an antiseptic such as iodine or 40–70 per cent alcohol (gin, whisky and vodka contain about 40 per cent)
- seek medical attention, preferably within 24 hours
- medical attention may include wound toilet, antimicrobial therapy, immunisation with tetanus toxoid and, if the bite occurred in a rabies endemic area, rabies post-exposure prophylaxis (whether or not pre-exposure prophylaxis was given).

12.2   Snake bites

Dangerous species of snakes are found in many tropical countries and local inhabitants are not infrequently bitten and even killed. Foreign travellers are rarely bitten.

12.2.1 Prevention

Snakes do not attack humans without provocation; they should never be disturbed, cornered, attacked or handled even if they are said to be harmless or appear to be dead. Walking barefoot in vegetation, swimming in murky estuaries or rivers matted with vegetation, and climbing trees or rocks covered with foliage are all risky. A light should be used at night.

12.2.2 Treatment

Travellers can be advised about first-aid measures:
- avoid tampering with the wound in any way
- immobilise the bitten limb with a splint or sling
- remove rings from a bitten hand
- transport the victim to a dispensary, health clinic or hospital as quickly as possible for immediate attention

Medical or hospital treatment will be assisted if a description of the snake is available. Antivenom treatment should only be administered by those experienced in its use.

12.3 Bites and stings by marine animals

Coelenterate (eg jellyfish, Portuguese man-o-war) stings can be inactivated with dilute acetic acid, eg vinegar, or sometimes baking soda. Adherent tentacles should be removed carefully (not with bare hands).

The excruciating pain of stinging fish (weevers, scorpionfish, stonefish, stingrays) may be relieved by immersing the limb in water at a temperature of about 45°C.

Sea urchin (Echinoderm) spines that get imbedded in the foot should be removed surgically after softening the skin with salicylic acid.

12.4 Hymenoptera stings (bees, wasps, hornets, ants)

People with known allergies to insect stings should carry emergency treatment (self-injectable 0.1 per cent adrenaline) and know how to use it. Even in a non-sensitised person, hundreds of stings by bees or wasps can be fatal through direct toxicity.

12.5 Scorpion stings and spider bites

The sting of most species of scorpion is painful. Some species in Mexico, North Africa, the Middle East, Latin America and India can cause myocardial damage and pancreatitis. Immediate medical help should be sought.

Very few species of spider are able to inject venom through human skin. Of those that can, a few species in South America and Australia cause neurotoxicity requiring specific antivenom treatment.

Spiders and scorpions may lurk in shoes and clothing, which should be checked before putting them on.

12.6 Leeches

Leeches are found in damp tropical forests and undergrowth. Wearing long socks, long trousers and boots liberally treated with repellants such as diethyltolumide helps to prevent them attaching to skin.

13 Medical considerations for the journey: travel by air, sea or land

13.1 Assessment of fitness to fly

Some guidelines on assessing fitness to fly are given below. However, different airlines have their own rules which can be checked with their medical adviser. A form (MEDIF) from the airline or travel agent should be completed by passenger and GP for any passenger with a relevant medical condition.

In general those with stable cardiac or respiratory conditions who can climb 12 stairs and walk 50 metres on the level without severe breathlessness or developing angina are fit to fly on commercial aeroplanes.

Those usually considered unsuitable for flying include those:
- markedly dyspnoeic at rest;
- with poorly controlled heart failure;
- with uncontrolled arrhythmias;
- with unstable angina;
- with a haemoglobin below 7.5 g/dl;
- with an infectious disease transmissible to other passengers;
- patients with a psychotic illness, unless stable and escorted.

Poorly controlled epileptics may need an increase in medication. Pregnant women should not travel after 36 weeks, and a letter stating their expected date of delivery and that they are fit to fly is desirable from 28 weeks.

Flying will usually need to be delayed for at least ten days after chest or abdominal surgery (even keyhole), and after a GI bleed, an uncomplicated myocardial infarction or a cerebrovascular accident with good recovery. It is advisable to wait 24 hours after a plaster cast is applied before a flight of under two hours and 48 hours if the flight is longer (or bivalve the plaster). Neonates should be at least 48 hours, and preferably at least two weeks, old before flying.

Facilities which may be available for pre booking for air travel
Equipment such as wheelchairs or other transport will be available within the airport and preboarding may be possible. On the plane a seat near the lavatory, an extra seat if necessary for a plaster cast (though the seat will have to be paid for), special dietary requirements and supplementary oxygen can be requested.

All travellers with pre-existing medical conditions are advised to declare their diagnosis to the insurance company and to carry their medication in their hand luggage with a separate note of its generic name and the dose.

13.2 Deep vein thrombosis

Any travel involving prolonged immobilisation, by land or air, can result in a deep vein thrombosis (DVT) with the risk of pulmonary embolus (PE). Those at increased risk include people with a history of thromboembolic disease, women taking an oral contraceptive or who are pregnant, those recently hospitalised, especially following major surgery, the obese, some patients with congestive heart failure, people with paralysis of the lower limbs and people with malignant disease. Dehydration may increase the risk.

Periodic flexion and extension exercises of the lower limbs, deep breathing exercises and walking around where feasible, are advised to help reduce the risk. People on long haul flights should also be advised to drink plenty of water and avoid excess coffee or alcohol. Those who are considered to be particularly at risk of DVT or PE need expert medical advice for the journey. Elastic support stockings, low dose aspirin, or anticoagulants (warfarin or low molecular weight heparin) may be prescribed.

13.3 Cruises

Those with pre-existing medical conditions may be considered more suitable for cruising than flying. This may exclude cruises involving a flight to join the ship. Medical facilities on board vary and travellers should be advised to enquire before they book. They should also realise that occasionally those with an acute medical emergency may have to disembark at whatever port is nearest whilst repatriation is arranged.

Rough weather may induce sea sickness. Although motion sickness is less likely on a larger ship, in some itineraries transfers may be necessary from the cruise ship to smaller vessels in order to go ashore. These may also require more agility and injuries have occurred.

Whilst eating and drinking on board is often considered safer than onshore, outbreaks of gastrointestinal infections or respiratory tract infections including influenza have occasionally occurred on board.

13.4 Jet lag

Long distance travel by land, sea or air can expose the traveller to tiring, crowded and stressful conditions with variable availability and suitability of meals and opportunities to sleep. When air travel crosses many time zones, additional symptoms on arrival can be caused by a lack of physiological adaptation to the local time.

Individuals are affected to varying degrees, increasing with the number of time zones crossed and tending to increase with advancing age. Adaptation to eastward travel generally takes longer than westwards.

Many proposed 'jet lag' regimens have little proof of efficacy but travellers can be advised to sleep/nap on flights to reduce the sleep debt and keep hydrated with plenty of water. A flight which arrives shortly before the local bedtime can be helpful. A few days acclimatisation to the new time zone should be allowed where performance of skilled tasks is important.

Research is being conducted into the careful timing of exposure to bright light, timing of meals and caffeine intake, exercise, sleep and naps. Research into the use of melatonin is also being undertaken. Melatonin is a pineal hormone which aids the circadian rhythm to shift to sleep/night mode. There are no long term toxicity studies. It is unlicensed in the UK and not reccommended for routine use at present.

Travellers with pre-existing medical conditions

14.1 Travellers with any pre-existing medical condition

Holiday destinations should be chosen and decisions to visit friends and relatives, or travel on business, taken with regard to fitness for travel, likely health risks and medical facilities at the destinations. Travellers should allow adequate time for medical preparation for such trips.

Travel medical insurance companies need to be aware of the medical conditions when the policy is obtained.

The traveller should carry a medical letter containing details of the condition or at least a list of any drug therapy with generic names and dosages. Any medication should be carried in hand luggage, or, preferably, divided between that of the traveller and a companion.

14.2 Additional notes on travel with certain conditions

14.2.1 Type 1 diabetes (Insulin dependent diabetes)

- diabetic meals for air travel can be ordered but are not considered necessary.
- for long haul east or west flights, instruction should be given on how to adjust insulin requirements during flight .
- sufficient insulin needs to be carried in a cool box in hand luggage. It should not be allowed to become frozen eg if in aircraft hold.
- injecting equipment and disposal method, blood monitoring equipment and test strips should be carried.
- instruction should be given on regular monitoring whilst travelling and especially in case of illness.
- advise to include snacks (eg cereal bars, biscuits, unsweetened fruit juice, sandwiches, glucose tablets etc) in hand luggage.
- those who have poor warning signs of hypoglycaemia are advised to travel with a companion trained in early recognition of hypo or hyperglycaemia.
- identification as a diabetic eg diabetic card or inscribed bracelet or medical letter should be carried at all times.
- advise on prevention of travel infections, especially skin and gastrointestinal, and consider whether a course of antibiotics should be carried.
- remind about the importance of keeping hydrated with plenty of non-alcoholic drinks in hot climates and the increased difficulty of early recognition of hypo and hyperglycaemia in such situations.

- hot climates increase susceptibility to hypoglycaemia. Diabetics may need to decrease insulin dose on arrival and monitor blood glucose more closely.
- Diabetes UK supplies useful information on many destinations, insulin type availability etc (see useful addresses).

14.2.2 Immunocompromised travellers (see below for additional notes on HIV infected travellers)

- live vaccines (yellow fever, oral typhoid, oral polio, BCG) should be avoided (see 8.3 and *Immunisation against Infectious Disease*).
- yellow fever infected areas should be avoided or the risk of travel without yellow fever protection should be assessed. In some cases the wisdom of travel may be questioned. Precautions should be advised to reduce mosquito bites dawn to dusk ie day biting mosquitoes (see 7.5).
- an exemption from yellow fever vaccination on medical grounds may be issued. Such letters are usually acceptable for entry directly from the UK, however they are less likely to be acceptable for travel between several different countries within the yellow fever zones. Although the advice to check with embassies may be given, in practice there is no absolute guarantee of acceptance in every situation overseas.
- inactivated vaccines can be administered although efficacy may be reduced.
- consider whether a course of early treatment antibiotics should be carried.

14.2.3 Additional information for HIV infected travellers

In addition to the advice given for immunocompromised travellers above:
- some countries require evidence of a negative HIV test as an entry requirement for certain categories of visitors, usually long-term visitors or students. Information is available from the Foreign and Commonwealth Office but these arrangements are liable to change and should be checked with the Embassy of the country concerned.
- inactivated vaccines should be administered as required but could be less effective, especially in those with a low CD4 lymphocyte count.
- vaccines may be more effective in those with higher CD4 counts who are taking anti-retroviral therapy. Although increases in viral load have been shown after administration of certain vaccines, these are generally thought to be transient and not clinically significant.
- MMR vaccine, a live vaccine, has been used safely in HIV infected individuals (see *Immunisation against Infectious Disease*) and may be appropriate for travellers going to regions where the risk of measles may be increased.
- yellow fever vaccination should be avoided as for other immunocompromised travellers (see above) on theoretical grounds. There is a lack of safety and efficacy data in HIV infected recipients, and this should be explained to asymptomatic HIV infected individuals who are determined to visit yellow fever risk areas whilst assessing the comparative risks of travelling with or without vaccine. A yellow fever waiver letter may be issued.

- the risk of opportunistic infections in HIV infected travellers may be increased (eg cryptosporidial diarrhoea). Advice about food and water hygiene should be offered, and patients may wish to carry antibiotics for rapid treatment (until they receive medical advice) or occasionally for prophylaxis.
- travellers intending to visit countries where TB prevalence is high, may be at increased risk of acquiring tuberculosis. Isoniazid chemoprophylaxis may be considered for those intending to stay for long periods.
- there are few data regarding interactions between anti-retroviral drugs and malaria chemoprophylaxis. One study has shown that mefloquine reduces protease inhibitor levels and it is possible that protease inhibitors could increase the blood levels of mefloquine and quinine. The clinical significance of this is, however, unclear. Mefloquine should probably not be offered to HIV infected travellers until more information is available. There are no reports of adverse interactions between chloroquine, proguanil or doxycycline and anti-retroviral drugs.

14.2.4 Splenectomised/asplenic travellers

- asplenic individuals are at increased risk of certain bacterial infections – pneumococcal, Hib and meningococcal C conjugate vaccines should be considered routinely. Meningococcal A&C or quadrivalent vaccine should be advised for travel to any suspected risk area.
- flu vaccine is recommended annually.
- risk from malaria is increased: high risk areas should be avoided if at all possible and meticulous care taken over prophylaxis.
- risk from babesiosis* is increased.
- check whether immunocompromised due to underlying condition (if so, see above).
- consider antibiotic prophylaxis (penicillin V, amoxycillin or erythromycin) or as immediate standby treatment to be taken if symptoms develop (pyrexia, malaise or shivering) until medical help is obtained.

*Babesiosis is caused by a protozoan parasite transmitted by ticks. It occurs in the north eastern coastal region of USA plus Wisconsin and sporadically in California and Georgia; also some areas of Europe. Prevention is by tick avoidance measures (see 7.5).

Pregnancy and travel

15.1 Introduction

Medical opinion is often sought as to whether overseas travel is safe during pregnancy, often in the hope of receiving reassurance that the risks are small.

While most pregnant women will enjoy a trouble-free journey, a pregnancy can never be guaranteed to be medically uneventful. Should medical treatment be required, there are likely to be advantages in being at home. Concerns overseas include the availability of medical expertise, possible lack of sterile equipment and blood, the absence of a doctor familiar with the individual history, language difficulties, and cost.

Some infectious diseases (eg malaria – see below) can be more severe during pregnancy and the wisdom of travel to infected areas should be questioned.

15.2 Malaria chemoprophylaxis

Malaria in pregnancy is usually a more severe disease which can result in abortion or stillbirth and complications in the mother.

All pregnant woman travelling to malarious regions should use chemoprophylaxis. Chloroquine and proguanil have a proven safety record in pregnancy. Mefloquine is not routinely used in pregnancy. The product data sheet states that in the absence of clinical experience, prophylactic use during pregnancy should be avoided as a matter of principle. Recent studies suggest that it is safe in the second and third trimesters. So, where a pregnant traveller cannot be dissuaded from visiting areas with a significant risk of highly chloroquine resistant *P.falciparum* malaria, it can be used cautiously in the second and third trimesters. Ongoing studies suggest it may also be safe in the first trimester. All fertile women using mefloquine should use reliable contraceptives, until three months after the last dose.

As always, chemoprophylactic drugs should be used in combination with measures to reduce mosquito bites. However, DEET-containing repellents should be used sparingly.

15.3 Travel immunisations

All vaccines should be avoided as far as possible in pregnancy because of the theoretical risk of damage to the developing fetus. Published data are generally not available.

For inactivated vaccines, the threat of the disease should be weighed against any risk of the vaccine. If post-exposure rabies immunisation is required, human diploid cell rabies vaccine should be advised.

Live vaccines should especially be avoided if possible. If a yellow fever vaccination certificate is required purely for entry purposes, a certificate of exemption will normally suffice. If the vaccine is inadvertently given to a pregnant woman, she should be reassured that neither yellow fever, nor oral polio or rubella vaccines, have been shown to cause fetal damage. If the danger of infection cannot be avoided, these vaccines could be administered. BCG is similarly best avoided during pregnancy although there is no evidence of harm.

Where the decision has been made to administer a vaccine, it should ideally be delayed until the second or third trimester of pregnancy.

15.4   Flying

Where travel is planned during pregnancy, 18–24 weeks is probably the ideal time. Airlines usually allow travel up to the 36th week, but after the 28th week a doctor's letter may be required stating that the pregnancy is normal, the expected delivery date, and that the doctor is happy for the woman to fly. The policy of individual airlines should be checked.

15.5   Travel medical insurance

Insurance policies should be checked for exclusions.

16 Travel with children

16.1 Introduction

Children differ from older travellers in their vaccine requirements, and in the medical problems they encounter. An ill child may compromise travel. Careful planning of all journeys is necessary to be prepared for likely emergencies.

16.2 Motion sickness

This is unusual in children under two years but frequent in 3–12 year olds. Being able to see the horizon and other external views helps to reduce the problem. Promethazine (Phenergan) can be used to reduce travel-associated nausea.

16.3 Respiratory tract infections

Throat and ear infections, especially sepsis in the middle ear, can prevent equilibration of pressure in the middle ear making children particularly susceptible to severe pain and discomfort when changing altitude. Flying may sometimes have to be delayed.

16.4 Diarrhoea

Acute diarrhoea in infants and young children creates a number of problems for travelling parents. Availability of clean nappies and the disposal of soiled material can be a logistic nightmare. Oral rehydration therapy is the most important therapy for a sick child and should always be carried. If the child is febrile, medical assistance should be sought.

16.5 Diet

Baby foods are often unavailable, or very expensive, in tropical countries and cows' milk may not be available. Only commercially bottled milk with a clear expiry date should be used. Dairy products are a common cause of diarrhoea in hot climates.

16.6 Skin problems

Nappy rash, prickly heat and sunburn occur frequently in hot, humid climates. Young children should be kept well-protected from the sun at all times, and given plenty of fluids. Soothing skin creams are a necessary requisite. Infection from a number of soil parasites through bare feet is a significant risk; children should be encouraged to wear shoes.

16.7 Medications

Enough medication for the whole journey should be provided for a child with an underlying medical problem. It is also wise to pack children's analgesics, oral replacement salts (see 5.3) and skin creams as these may not be readily available.

17.1 Introduction

The fear of tropical illness often worries those who have spent some time in the tropics, and many returnees express concern about harbouring diseases which may lead to health problems later in life. Even those who have had little illness during their stay are often keen to undergo screening on their return.

17.2 Screening asymptomatic returnees

Post-tropical screening is reassuring to the recipient and does produce a significant number of abnormal results. In most cases it can be done by the general practitioner, relatively few requiring referral to a specialist tropical diseases unit.

In one study, one in four asymptomatic people returning from at least three months in the tropics had an abnormality detected on screening. Three quarters of these were parasitic gut infections identified by **stool examination** for cysts, ova and parasites. **Schistosomal serology** was positive in nearly 11 per cent of those who had visited schistosomal areas, whether or not they gave a history of exposure. About eight per cent had an eosinophilia on the blood count, and further investigation resulted in a relevant tropical diagnosis in 40 per cent of these. Physical examination was of limited use in detecting tropical illness in these returnees, but picked up some non-tropical pathology. The yield from additional tests was small. Screening for schistosomiasis is recommended for all those who may have been exposed, even if asymptomatic. This should include schistosome ELISA and eosinophil count, and also microscopy of stool and terminal urine. Screening should start at least 12 weeks after exposure to allow time for seroconversion.

17.3 Investigation of symptomatic returnees

Management of those returning with symptoms depends on the nature of the problem, but many tropical diseases are best handled by a specialised tropical diseases unit where the necessary further investigations can be done and where there is access to a laboratory familiar with the tests involved. The incidence of individual diseases in tropical countries may change from year to year as epidemics occur and the last few years have seen notable instances of new or resurgent infections arising in the tropics. Tropical specialists are also more likely to be able to identify tropical skin diseases which may be unfamiliar to UK-based dermatologists. The travel history should be included on microbiology request forms, as unusual antimicrobial resistance patterns may occur.

17.3.1 Fever

The differential diagnosis of fever includes imported disease as well as conditions prevalent in the UK. Malaria must be excluded as a matter of urgency in all cases of febrile illness in those who have visited malaria endemic areas. (Malaria is a great mimic and should be considered in **any** patient who is unwell and has potentially been exposed.) **Thick and thin blood films** should be prepared without delay. Most cases of *Plasmodium falciparum* malaria imported into the UK present within the first three months, but presentation can be delayed for up to one year. Longer intervals have been recorded for the relapsing forms of malaria.

Enteric fever, dengue, pneumonia (including legionnaires' disease and other atypical pneumonias), hepatitis and acute schistosomiasis (Katayama fever) should also be considered. Early advice should be sought from a physician experienced in tropical and infectious diseases if the diagnosis is unclear.

17.3.2 Diarrhoea

Diarrhoea is frequent among returning travellers and many do not seek medical attention. A careful history is essential for correct diagnosis and should include a travel history, the time elapsed since returning to the UK and the duration of diarrhoea. This information should be included on the laboratory request form accompanying **stool microscopy and culture**.

Travellers' diarrhoea usually occurs during travel or very shortly after returning home. The longer the history, the more likely is a parasitic (eg *Giardia*, *Entamoeba histolytica*, *Cyclospora*) rather than a bacterial or viral cause. It should always be borne in mind that malaria can present as a diarrhoeal illness.

17.3.3 Pharyngitis

Throat swabs from patients with pharyngitis should include the history of recent travel so that culture for *Corynebacterium diphtheriae* is included where appropriate. Lassa fever should be considered in cases of fever and pharyngitis from rural West Africa.

17.3.4 Hepatitis

Hepatitis A and B together account for most cases of imported viral hepatitis. Less commonly hepatitis C and E, coxiella, cytomegalovirus, glandular fever or toxoplasma may be responsible for a hepatic illness. Malaria can present as hepatitis.

17.3.5 HIV infection

Where appropriate, tactful discussion of potential risk factors for HIV exposure abroad should form part of a post-travel consultation.

17.3.6 Skin conditions

Skin infections, from all groups of infectious agent including insects, are common in the tropics. Dermatophyte infections frequently occur. Pitfalls include cutaneous diphtheria and cutaneous leishmaniasis. Myiasis may be mis-diagnosed as furunculosis.

17.3.7 Systemic parasitoses

Helminth infections, eg onchocerciasis, loiasis, may present long after the patient has returned to the UK. Schistosomiasis may present acutely a few weeks or months after exposure, but presentation can be long-delayed and, in the case of genito-urinary involvement, may be overlooked or misdiagnosed.

References

Behrens RH, Colins M, Botto B, Heptonstall J. 'Risk for British travellers of acquiring hepatitis A' *BMJ* 1995; **311:** 193.

Bonington A, Hardbord M, Davidson RN, Cropley I, Behrens RH. 'Immunisation against Japanese encephalitis' *Lancet* 1995; **345:** 1445–6.

Bradley DJ and Bannister B. 'Guidelines for malaria prevention in travellers from the United Kingdom for 2001' *Commun. Dis and Pub. Health* 2001; **4:** 84–101.

Goodyer L, Behrens RH. Short report: 'The safety and toxicity of insect repellents' *Am J Trop Med Hyg* 1998; **59 (2):** 323–4.

Hargarten SW, Baker TD, Guptill K. 'Overseas fatalities of the united States citizen travellers: an analysis of deaths related to international travellers' *Ann Emerg Med* 1991; **20:** 622-6.

Phillips-Howard PA, Steffen R, Kerr L, Vanhauwere B, Schildknecht J, Fuchs E, Edwards R. 'Safety of mefloquine and other antimalarial agents in the first trimester of pregnancy' *J Travel Med* 1998; **5:** 121–6.

Sagliocca L, Amoroso P, Stroffolini T, *et al.* 'Efficacy of hepatitis A vaccine in prevention of secondary hepatitis A infection: a randomised trial' *Lancet* 1999; **353:** 1136–9.

Shanks GD, Kremsner PG, Sukwa TY, Van der Berg JD, Shapiro TA. Scott TR, Chulay JD. 'Atovaquone and proguanil hydrochloride for prophylaxis of malaria' *J Travel Med* 1999; **6(suppl1):** 121–6.

Steffen R, Rickenbach M, Willhelm U, *et al.* 'Health problems after travel to developing countries' *J Infect Dis* 1987; **156:** 84–91.

Tsai T. 'Inactivated Japanese encephalitis virus vaccine; Recommendations of the Advisory Committee on Immunisation Practices (ACIP)' *MMWR* 1993; **42(RR-1):** 1–15.

Zuckerman J, Kirkpatrick C, Huang M. 'Immunogenicity and reactogenicity of Avaxim (160AU) as compared with Havrix (1440 EL.U) as a booster following primary immunisation with Havrix (1440 EL. U) against hepatitis A' *J Travel Med* 1998; **5:** 18–22.

Publications – written for Health Professionals

Immunisation against Infectious Disease, UK Departments of Health, 1996. London: HMSO (New edition due 2001/02).

International Travel and Health. Vaccination Requirements and Health Advice, Geneva: World Health Organization 2001 (revised annually).

Lockie C, Walker E, Calvert L *et al* (Eds) *Travel Medicine and Migrant Health,* Harcourt Publishers Ltd, 2000.

Benenson A. *Control of Communicable Diseases Manual* 1995. An offical report of the American Public Health Association, Washington.

Behrens RH, McAdam KPWJ (Eds). 'Travel Medicine' *British Medical Bulletin* 1993; **49** No2. Churchill Livingstone, 1993.

Walker E, Williams G, Raeside F. *ABC of Healthy Travel,* BMJ Books, 1993.

Bell D, *Lecture Notes on Tropical Medicine,* Blackwell Scientific Publications.

Cook ed. *Manson's Tropical Diseases,* Saunders Company Ltd, 1996.

Kassianos GC. *Immunisation: Childhood and Travel Health,* Blackwell Science, 2000 (in press).

Pollard AJ, Murdoch DR. *The High Altitude Medicine Handbook,* Radcliffe Medical Press, Oxford and New York 1997.

The Royal Geographical Society. *Expedition Medicine,* Profile Books 1998.

Department of Health. *Memorandum on Rabies. Prevention and Control,* February 2000.

Takahashi H, Pool V, Tsai F, Chen RT. *Adverse Events After Japanese Encephalitis Vaccination,* Vaccine 18 (2000); 2963–2969.

Confavreux C, Suissa S, Saddier P, Bourdes V, Vukusic S. 'Vaccinations and the Risk of Disease in Multiple Sclerosis', *N Eng J Med* 2001; **344:** 319–26.

Webster G, Barnes E, Dusheiko G, Franklin I. 'Protecting Travellers from Hepatitis A', *BMJ* 2001; **322** 1194–5.

Publications – written for travellers/non-medical persons

Bedford H, Elliman D. *Childhood immunisation: a review for parents and carers,* Health Education Authority, 1998.

Dawood R. *Travellers Health: How to stay healthy abroad,* Oxford University Press, 1992.

Department of Health. *Health Advice for Travellers* (T6).
Single copies can be ordered, free of charge, on the Health Literature line, 0800 555 777.

Bulk copies (more than 10) must be ordered from
Department of Health
PO Box 777
London SE1 6XH
Fax: 01623 724524
Email: doh@prolog.uk.com
The information in this booklet is available and regulary updated on the computerised data service PRESTEL.

Lankaster T. *Good health good travel*, Hodder and Stoughton Ltd, London, 1995.

Lea G, Carroll B. *Understanding Travel and Holiday Health*, Family Doctor Series. The British Medical Association, 1997.

'Lonely Planet' series. Healthy travel:
Asia and India
Central and South America
Australia, NZ and the Pacific.

Wilson-Howarth J. *Bugs, Bites and Bowels*, Cadogan Guides, London, 1999.

Wilson-Howarth J, Elis M. *Your Child's Health Abroad. A manual for travelling parents*, Bradt Publications, UK, 1998.

Appendix 1:
Exemption from the requirement for an International Certificate of Vaccination

Where a physician advises that an adult, or infant, should not be vaccinated on medical grounds this should be written on headed writing paper which will be taken into consideration by the port health authorities in the destination country. The advice has often been given to check the acceptability with the UK Embassy or High Commission of that country, although in practice not all Embassies are able to guarantee the attitude of individual port health officials. However if the Embassy provides a letter accepting the exemption certificate this could be helpful on entry.

Example

Re: Name _____

Address _____

_____

_____

_____

This is to certify that on medical grounds I advise that _____ vaccine is contraindicated in the above named person and should not therefore be given.

Date _____

Signed _____

Print name _____

(PRACTICE STAMP)

Appendix 2:
Useful addresses and telephone numbers

Consultant in Communicable Disease Control

Name_____

Tel No. _____

(please insert details of your local CCDC)

Telephone advice lines for health professionals
(Calls from the public cannot be answered by these services – please do not give these numbers out to patients)

Public Health Laboratory Service (PHLS)
Communicable Disease Surveillance Centre (CDSC)
Travel Medicine Unit
61 Colindale Avenue, London NW9 5EQ
Tel: 020 8200 6868   Service open weekdays 10am–12 midday

PHLS Malaria Reference Laboratory
London School of Hygiene and Tropical Medicine
Keppel Street, London WC1E 7HT
Tel: 020 7636 3924   Service open 9am–4.30pm

Travel Medicine Division of Scottish Centre for Infection and Environmental Health (SCIEH)
Clifton House, Clifton Place
Glasgow G3 7LN
For professional users of Travax only:
Tel: 0141 300 1130   Service open weekdays 2–4pm

Hospital for Tropical Diseases Travel Clinic
Mortimer Market Centre, Capper Street
off Tottenham Court Road
London WC1E 6AU
Tel: 020 7387 9600

Department of Infection & Tropical Medicine
Northwick Park Hospital, Harrow HA1 3UJ
Tel: 020 8869 2831

Department of Infection and Tropical Medicine
Birmingham Heartlands Hospital
Birmingham B9 5ST
Tel: 0121 766 6611 ext 4403/4382/4535

John Warin Ward
The Churchill Hospital
Headington
Oxford OX3 7LJ
Tel: 01865 225214

Liverpool School of Tropical Medicine
Pembroke Place
Liverpool L3 5QA
Tel: 0151 708 9393

Department of Infectious Diseases and Tropical Medicine
North Manchester General Hospital
Delaunays Road
Manchester M8 5RB
Tel: 0161 720 2677

Data bases/'On Line' travel advice
Travax – Scottish Centre for Infection and Environmental Health website for health care professionals (continually updated – registration is on-line at www.axl.co.uk/scieh)

Fit for travel – NHS website for the public consistent with Travax at www.fitfortravel.scot.nhs.uk

TRAVELLER: database with monthly updates
Enquiries to Travellers Direct Ltd, Tel 0114 282 3488

Advice paylines available to the public
(Limited to recorded messages)

Malaria Reference Laboratory   Tel: 0891 600350

Hospital for Tropical Diseases   Tel: 09061 337733

Liverpool School of Tropical Medicine Tel: 0891 172111

MASTA (Medical Advisory Service
for Travellers Abroad)   Tel: 0891 224100

Other useful telephone numbers

British Diabetic Association   Tel: 020 7323 1531

Department of Health (for publications)   Tel: 0800 555777

Foreign and Commonwealth Office   Tel: 020 7270 4129

Medic - Alert Foundation   Tel: 020 7833 3034

National AIDS Helpline   Tel: 0800 567123

Vaccine manufacturers and distributors

Aventis Pasteur MSD
northern areas of the country   Tel: 0321 1822 2463
southern areas of the country   Tel: 0321 2822 2463

Baxter Hyland Immuno   Tel: 01635 206265

Celltech Medeva   Tel: 01372 364000

Farillon   Tel: 01708 379000

MASTA   Tel: 0113 2387500

GlaxoSmithKline
enquiries   Tel: 0808 100 2228
orders   Tel: 0808 100 9997

Other useful web site addresses

www.phls.co.uk
Web site of the Public Health Laboratory Service. Has access to CDR reports and
various facts and figures.

www.fco.gov.uk/
Foreign and Commonwealth Office

www.who.int/index.html
World Health Organization

www.who.int/wer/
Weekly Epidemiology Record (WER) produced by WHO.

www.who.int/emc/outbreak_news/index.html
Web site of Emerging and other Communicable Diseases Surveillance and Control (EMC) – outbreak news, disease information and surveillance.

www.cdc.gov
Web site of the Centre for Disease Control and Prevention (USA), which includes access to MMWR and various data and statistics.

www.istm.org
Web site of the International Society of Travel Medicine, which includes access to Journal of Travel Medicine.

Index of countries

Comments on the publication

Comments, corrections and suggestions for improving future editions of this publication, including information from readers who have up to date knowledge of a particular overseas area, are welcome, either by letter, email or on this sheet.

Please make notes below (including the date to which the information refers):

Signed _____

Name _____

Address _____

_____

_____

_____

Please return to:
Dr Jane Leese
Department of Health
Room 605A
Skipton House
80 London Road
London SE1 6LH

Email: jane.leese@doh.gsi.gov.uk

Notes

Notes

Notes

Notes

Notes

Notes